Cognitive Behaviour Therapy for Social Anxiety

A CBT workbook to help you overcome symptoms of social anxiety and cope better with social situations

Written by Dr James Manning, ClinPsyD

Cognitive Behaviour Therapy for Social Anxiety: A CBT Workbook to help you overcome symptoms of social anxiety and cope better with social situations

Written by

Dr James Manning, ClinPsyD

Published by

Ridgeman Mental Health Books

This edition printed 2024

ISBN - 9781917369138

Limits of liability/disclaimer of warranty –

The author does not take responsibility for any possible consequences from any treatment, procedure, test exercise or action of any person reading or following the information in this book. The publication of this book does not constitute the practice of medicine and this book does not attempt to replace any other instructions from your doctor or qualified practitioner. The author advises the reader to check with a doctor or qualified practitioner before undertaking any course of treatment.

Whilst the author has used his best efforts in preparing this book, the makes no representations or warranties with respect to the accuracy or the completeness of the contents of this book and specifically disclaim any implied warranties or merchantability or fitness for a particular purpose. No warranty may be created or extended. The advice and strategies contained herein may not be suitable for your situation. You should where necessary consult with a professional where appropriate.

*****A PDF link to print out this book is located at the end of Chapter 16 in the chapter summary section.**

The authors shall not be liable for any loss or profit or any other commercial damages, including but not limited to special, incidental, consequential or other damages.

Case examples referred to in this book are generic and based on collective presentations. No relation to any specific person is either implied or intended.

About the author

Dr James Manning is a Consultant Clinical Psychologist. James has post-graduate qualifications in both Clinical Psychology and Counselling Psychology. He has regularly offered workshops and training to clinicians throughout the United Kingdom on Cognitive Behaviour Therapy and continues to work as a practicing psychologist.

Also by Dr James Manning

Think About Your Thinking to Stop Depression

How to Help Your Loved One Overcome Depression

CBT for Panic

CBT Worksheets

CBT: What it is and how it works (2nd Edition)

My CBT Journal

The Little Book on CBT for Anxiety

CBT Worksheets for Anxiety

CBT Worksheets for Teenage Social Anxiety

A Journey with Panic

The misunderstood dog

Contents

1 What is social anxiety?

You are probably reading this book because either you or someone you know is suffering with social anxiety. No doubt, you are probably already aware just how disabling social anxiety can be. It can affect people from all areas of life, regardless of their wealth, education, intelligence, and social status. Social anxiety can have a huge impact on self-esteem, well-being and happiness. As well as this, it can disrupt relationships and get in the way of career progression. The consequence for the sufferer is often a sense of isolation, loneliness, and a lack of emotional connection with others, even if the individual is in a relationship or surrounded by others.

Social anxiety is a silent condition, often invisible to people who don't suffer from it. Many people are completely unaware that people they know very well suffer from social anxiety. This is due to the fact that individuals who suffer with social anxiety, are often so skilled at hiding it.

Sometimes the terms social anxiety and shyness are used inter-changeably. However, they are very different. People who are shy recognise they are shy, they don't try to hide it, unlike people with social anxiety.

Estimates vary amongst research papers published, but it is generally suggested that within 5% and 15% of Western individuals will suffer with social anxiety during some part of their lifetime.

The effects of social anxiety are not necessarily the same for all individuals. For some, their anxiety may be restricted to just one or two specific areas, for example, public speaking, whereas for others it surfaces in multiple life situations and has a wide impact on many areas of their social functioning. In our practice we have worked with large numbers of individuals with social anxiety and the most common anxiety provoking situations appear to be;

- Talking to strangers
- Attending functions where there is a large group of people (e.g., a dinner party)
- Meeting authority figures
- Being watched while completing an activity
- Being questioned in front of others
- Being introduced to others
- Public speaking

The most commonly reported symptoms of social anxiety tend to be a dry mouth, feeling light-headed, feeling nauseous, legs shaking, feeling hot, sweating, stomach cramps, feeling tight in the chest, heart racing, trembling, a lump in the throat, and the mind going blank (see figure 1.) When the above types of bodily processes occur many individuals with social anxiety monitor their symptoms or try to control their anxiety with a great deal of concern that others in their social group may notice that there is something not quite right with them. Individuals with social anxiety may then try to cover up their symptoms using some of the strategies listed below.

Commonly used strategies by people with social anxiety

- Focus on the self to imagine how the self might be coming across to others.
- Stand near a doorway or a window to reduce sweating.
- Wear makeup to mask redness in the face.
- Try to avoid eye-contact with other people.
- Try not to hold a glass in front of others to disguise shaking.
- Rehearse what to say before speaking.
- Keep a low profile and stay in the background for fear of doing something silly and drawing attention to the self.
- Stand next to somebody safe.
- Keep conversation to a bare minimum.
- Fill awkward silences in conversation.
- Drink alcohol to relax before going out.
- Expect the self to put on a performance to amuse others.
- Leave situations early wherever possible.
- Tell stories or jokes to entertain others.

Figure 1. What happens in the body with social anxiety

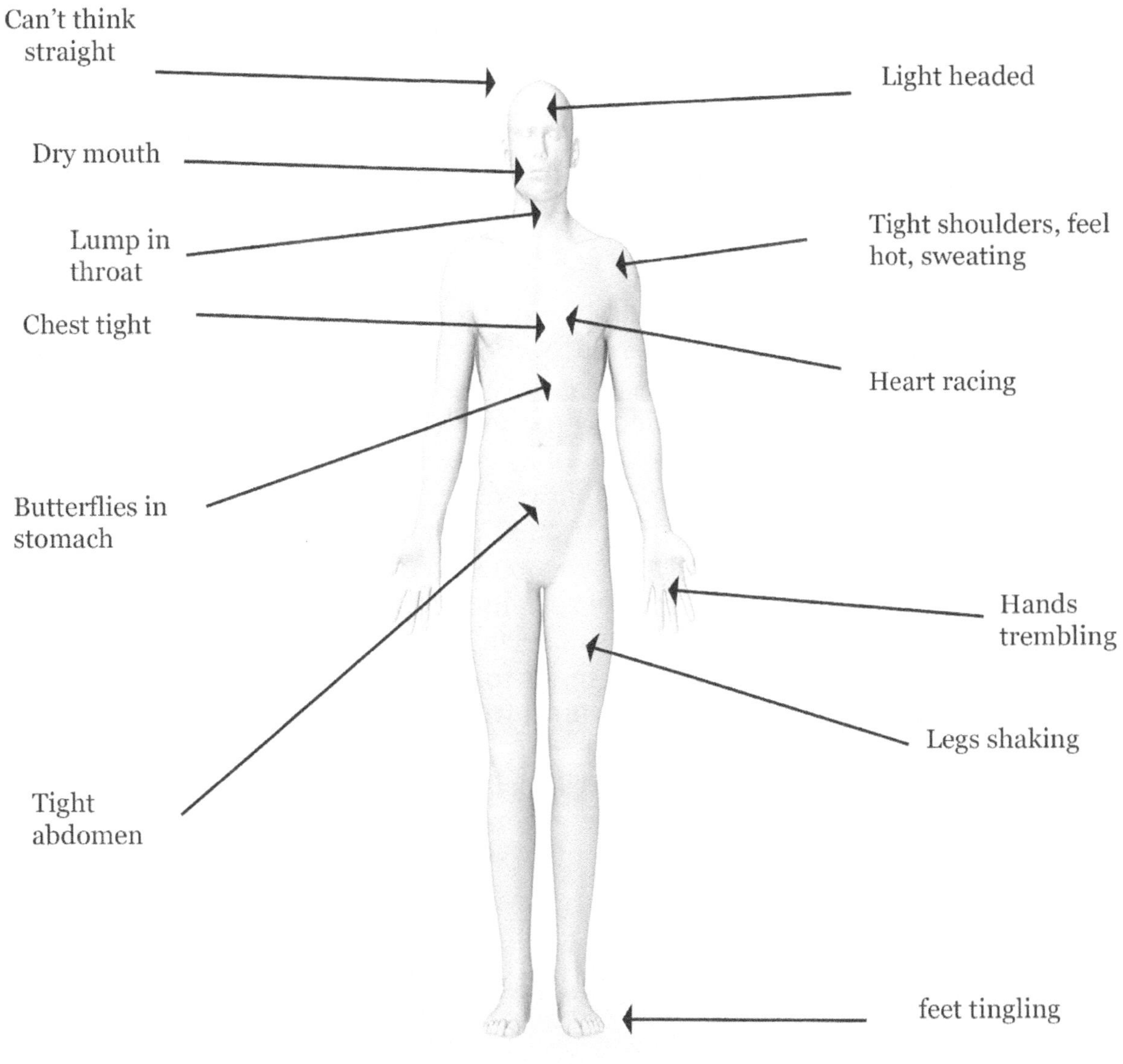

Chapter summary

What is social anxiety?

- Social anxiety is a form of anxiety that people experience when they are around other people.
- Social anxiety can occur to anybody, regardless of intelligence, attractiveness, social status, and wealth.
- Between 5 and 15% of the population suffer with social anxiety.
- People can feel socially anxious about different areas of social contact.
- Social anxiety tends to create a lot of physical symptoms, from a dry mouth to trembling limbs.
- Most people with social anxiety try to hide their anxiety from others using a range of different strategies.

2 The structure of the brain

In order to help you understand how social anxiety occurs I am going to simplify a highly complex neuro-biological process.

The brain

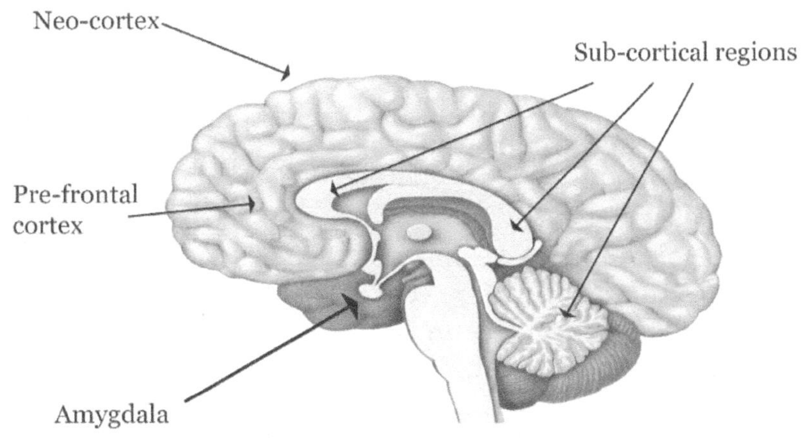

Figure 2. Structure of the brain

There are three main structures that it is advisable to know about to understand social anxiety. These areas are the neocortex, the prefrontal cortex, and the subcortical regions, see figure 2.

The neocortex

This is a part of the brain responsible for thinking, planning, and logical thought. We use this part of the brain to understand language, to make calculations, and to problem-solve. The neocortex is used quite a lot when we carry out complex thinking.

The prefrontal cortex

The prefrontal cortex is an essential part of the brain for psychological wellness. The prefrontal cortex's main job is to act as a communication system between the neocortex and the subcortical region. It has many important functions. It quietens down noise in the mind and it can call off emotional reactions. We also use this part of our brain to think about our thinking and to bring choices into conscious awareness. The prefrontal cortex is highly affected by social anxiety. This may result in you feeling that you are unable to think straight or to organise your thoughts.

The subcortical regions

The subcortical regions - which take their name because they are located underneath the brains outer cortex area - could be described as a primitive or animal brain, as we share similar brain structures with mammals. The subcortical regions' predominant interest is survival. Understandably, therefore, this is where our main pleasure and pain centres are located.

Subcortical regions of the brain become highly active when we experience perceived threat; whether real or imagined. When people become socially anxious, subcortical brain regions release neurochemicals known as **catecholamines** which improve the way that primitive brain regions function. In lay terms, catecholamines work a bit like a turbo-boost or a power-up for the animal brain. When primitive brain regions become more active, people become more aware of all of their senses. As a result of this, they may see, hear, feel, taste, and smell things more strongly (Guzman, Tronson, Jovasevic Sato, Guedea, Mizukami, Nishimori & Radulovic, 2013). Heightened sensory perception leads people to become much more aware of their bodily processes. For example, for some people with social their face may feel red hot, whereas to observers it is not really noticeable.

The impact of catecholamines

Many people with social anxiety experience mental clouding in social situations. This is due to the impact of catecholamines. Catecholamines although enhancing the effects of the subcortical region leach or spread into the nearby prefrontal cortex and stop it functioning effectively. This leaching effect is usually only temporary and when the threat dies down and neurochemicals are reabsorbed, the prefrontal cortex starts to work normally as before.

So, in summary, when you experience social anxiety it will be difficult for you to think straight and your mind will feel foggy. The neocortex is not able to function properly as to do this it needs the assistance of the prefrontal cortex to hold ideas in mind, and to think about thoughts at the at the same time. When the prefrontal cortex comes back on line again you will find that you are able to think clearly again once more.

Chapter summary
The structure of the brain

- The functioning of the brain can be separated into three main areas, the subcortical region, the prefrontal cortex, and the neocortex.
- The subcortical region takes care of our animal functions, the neocortex deals with our complex thinking, and the prefrontal cortex operates as a go between.
- The subcortical region becomes more dominant when we experience threat. The neocortex becomes more dominant when we are relaxed.

3 The brain's alarm system

In the middle of the subcortical regions of the brain lie our two amygdalae, see figure 3.

The brain

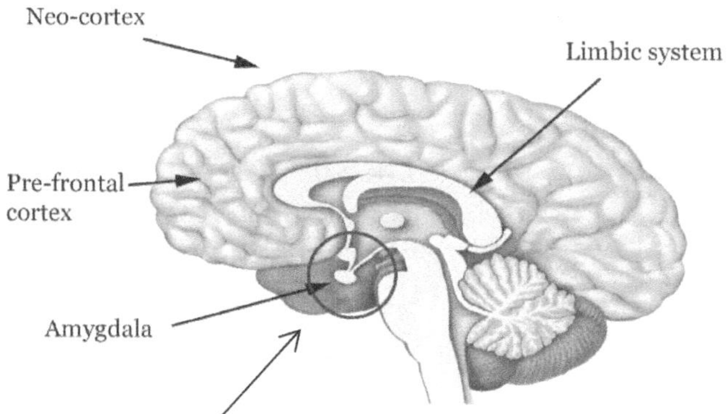

Figure 3. The location of the amygdala

> **The Threat Perception Centre**
>
> Research indicates that despite the small size of the amygdalae and the regions that surround it, this area of the brain has its own dedicated memory system which holds key information about past traumatic incidents (LeDoux, 2015). This memory system appears to operate like a lookout post or a sieve. It observes everything that passes through our senses and activates the amygdala if it notices any sensory stimuli that might be a slight match for past painful physical or psychological experiences. For simplicity I will refer to this memory system as the **'Threat Perception Centre.'**

I will illustrate how this process works with an example from my childhood. When I was around eight or nine I used to pick wild brambles and spent many hours enjoying myself looking for the largest, ripest berries to eat. One summer day I picked what I thought was the ultimate bramble and was just about to put it in my mouth when I became aware of a maggot wriggling in the stem and touching my lips. I immediately felt a wave of disgust ripple through my whole body. Practically every hair on my body stood on end as I immediately realised I could have eaten this maggot as well as others unknowingly. I instinctively threw the berry as far as I could away from me, then turned around and walked off.

After the above incident I developed an aversion to eating brambles, which progressed to supermarket berries, such as raspberries which had a similar shape, and then later to jams containing raspberries or blackberries. My body produced an automatic response to the cue of any fruit that was shaped anything like a blackberry. As a child I didn't stop to think about what was going on or to challenge my fears, I simply avoided eating these types of berries. I didn't view it as a problem, and to be honest it didn't affect my life very much.

My situation with berries is typical of processes that occur in the subcortical region of the brain. According to models of emotional intelligence
(Golman, 1997) the subcortical region, due to its more primitive nature puts a significant focus on survival. It also obtains access to information from the senses slightly before the neocortex. If while accessing sensory information it picks up cues associated with past painful or frightening events (trauma) it immediately triggers biological processes that generate defensive or offensive type reactions (i.e., the fight-flight response). Importantly, it will also do this before the rational mind has a chance to think about what action to take. I have drawn a hypothetical, simplified model of how this process occurs (see figure 4).

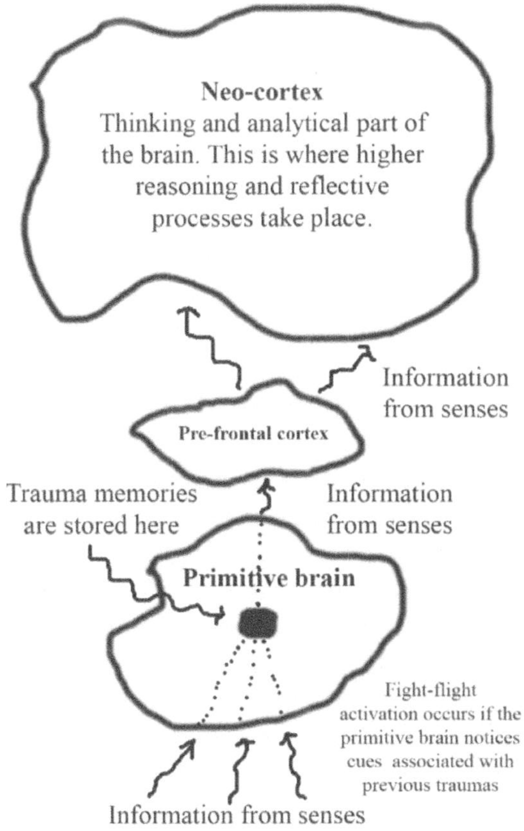

Figure 4. Model of the threat perception centre in action

At this point I am not going to go into great detail about the biology of the threat perception centre. If you are interested in finding out more about the biology of emotions you can read an excellent and highly readable review of this area within Daniel Goleman's book on Emotional Intelligence (1995). Early chapters in Goleman's book cover "Emotional Hijacking" whereas other areas within his book will help you understand how emotions work.

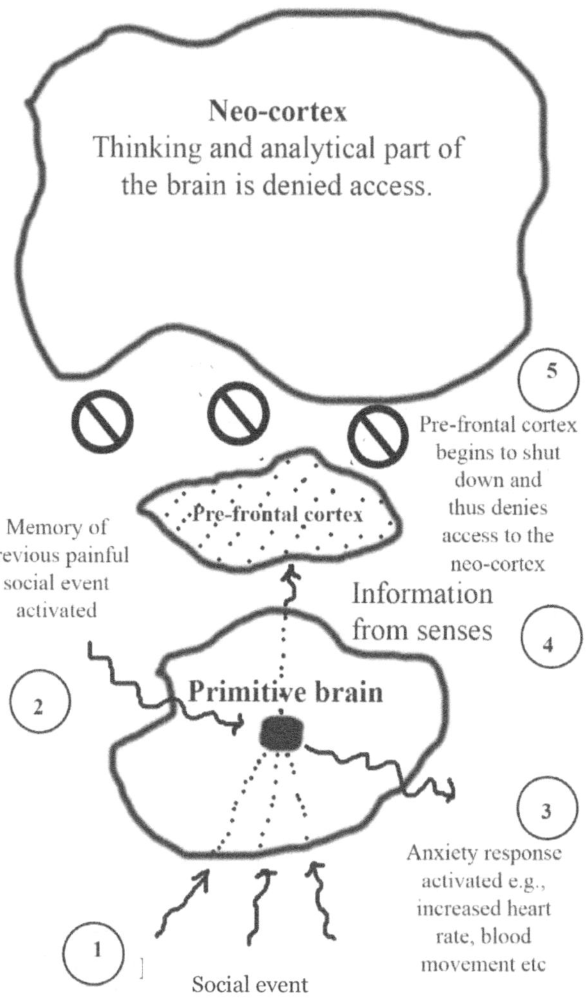

Figure 5. Social event and prepared response

When the subcortical mind is helpful

Most of us, if we think about it enough, will probably be able to remember situations where our subcortical mind has helped ourselves or others in tricky situations. Indeed, while I was thinking of ideas for this book I remembered a potentially life changing incident that I observed one hot summer weekend in Suffolk, England. My family had been invited to a barbeque at a friend's house. Many friends and colleagues had brought their children. The children were playing in the garden and the adults were caught up in conversation around the host's outdoor pool. At one point I heard one lady whisper "Has anybody seen Molly?" Immediately out of the corner of my eye I noticed a heavily pregnant colleague of mine jumping fully clothed into the pool and a second or so later pulling a two year old girl out of the pool **by her hair**. The incident happened in seconds, and the whole rescue operation occurred before the rest of us had time to think.

Chapter summary

The brain's alarm system

- The subcortical region of the brain helps the body to take immediate action in the face of perceived threat.
- When working effectively the subcortical region can literally be a life saver.
- The threat perception centre records traumatic incidents in its memory to warn the individual against future similar dangers.
- If past social events were traumatic, they can remain as unprocessed memories in the brain's threat perception centre. Similar events are then likely to trigger anxiety.

4 How does social anxiety start?

For many sufferers of social anxiety a typical question is "Why me?" Why do I become so anxious in social occasions while others around me appear so relaxed and confident? If you have asked yourself this type of question then you will find out as you read this chapter that there are a number of factors that are likely to be responsible for triggering social anxiety, some of which are more surprising than others.

A better memory for trauma

The most likely explanation that tells us why some of us feel more social anxiety than others is our genetic predisposition. For example, some of us have more sensitive oxytocin receptor sites in our brain. This can lead to enhanced encoding of childhood social memories, both positive and negative, (Yomayra & colleagues, 2013). Based on this hypothesis, individuals with more sensitive oxytocin receptors will encode traumatic social memories more strongly than those individuals with less sensitive receptor sites. As a result, individuals with stronger memory encoding will more readily notice environmental cues associated with past traumas. This in turn will lead to more frequent anxiety response activations in social situations.

Early traumatic incidents

As mentioned in the previous chapter another potential explanation for social anxiety is traumatic childhood experiences. At an early age individuals with social anxiety may have been exposed to more extreme social traumas than others. In this respect, it may just be a matter of chance that a child happens to end up in a classroom with a dysfunctional teacher or a socially challenging peer group. When you are a child it is very difficult to prevent yourself from being humiliated or ridiculed by a teacher in front of the whole class at school, being laughed at by other children in the class, being picked on for blushing etc. If you have experienced these types of situations then these incidents are easily encoded in the brains subcortical brain regions. This may lead to activation of the anxiety response in later situations which have similar cues (e.g., an authority figure asking you questions, being in a room full of people etc.) Bear in mind that the amount of time that has passed since the original incident is irrelevant. The threat perception centre does not recognise time. Activation can occur even though the original traumatic incidents may have happened years or even decades before.

We learn what to fear through interactions with care givers

According to research completed by Dr Jacek Debiec and Dr Reina Sullivan (2014) at the University of Michigan babies as young as a few days old can learn what to fear by detecting specific smells given off by their mother. A further suggestion by Dr Gina Mireaut of Johnson State College, is that babies from the age of six months continuously look to their care givers as a source of emotional information (or as an emotional reference point). Thus, when babies come across something unusual they look to their care giver to find out how to react. In this way they can discover what to fear, what to find humorous etc. A good example of this is demonstrated with research carried out with very small children below the age of two. Toddlers (pre-two years) who have not previously been exposed to snakes are placed in a room within which there is a large glass tank full of snakes. Generally, the children show a huge amount of curiously for these snakes. It is almost as though if it were possible to get their body into this tank full of snakes they would freely do it. The child is then removed but is allowed to watch their adult caregiver go into the same room. If the caregiver is seen by the child experiencing an aversive reaction to the snakes, and the child is placed in the room once more, instead of feeling curious as he or she did previously, the child becomes distressed and wants to return to his or her care-giver. The child instantaneously learns to fear snakes by watching the reaction of his/her caregiver. In this respect, we are programmed to associate fear with specific cues very quickly from a very early age. From an evolutionary perspective this type of process appears beneficial as quickly learning what to fear undoubtedly helps us to live longer. This then begs the question – Based on the above mentioned learning mechanism, what do young children learn if they witness their adult caregivers showing a fear reaction to an impending social situation?

Social Learning

As suggested above, the environment that we are brought up in can have a long lasting impact on our behaviour. This occurs as a result of the fact that as children we learn automatically through imitation. We do not realise that we are copying others, it just happens naturally. In this respect, if children are brought up in an environment where one or both parent figures have engaged in safety behaviours connected to social anxiety, then there is an increased probability that these children will engage in similar social habits as they grow up.

Core Beliefs

Notable researchers in the field of CBT, Professors Clark and Wells suggest in their model of social anxiety that specific social trigger situations activate core beliefs and assumptions such as "I am defective", "I am abnormal", "I am different", "I am weird" and "People don't like me." It is generally thought that these beliefs patterns are formed as a result of painful childhood experiences, and that these experiences lead children and adolescents to search for negative meanings about themselves, the world, and others.

Beliefs can also be formed as a result of interactions between the self and significant others (often care givers). This can happen in an obvious abusive way such as a parent stating "What's wrong with you... Why haven't you got any friends?" or in more subtle ways such as the parent limiting opportunities for their children to have social engagements for fear that they will be unable to cope, or telling their children to be quiet because people are watching. Beliefs will be covered in more detail in chapter 15.

Beliefs

All beliefs, positive or negative act like prejudices. Prejudices behave like self-fulfilling prophecies. We tend to seek out what we 'know', which is often inaccurate and limited.

Core beliefs can be thought of as fundamental meanings about the self, and the world that we believe to be unquestioningly true. It is quite easy to see how having a positive belief like "I am a likeable person" is more useful than negative beliefs such as "I am abnormal" and "I am unacceptable."

Chapter summary

How does social anxiety start?

- Some of us are genetically predisposed to remember traumatic social events more clearly than others.
- Some of us are exposed to more damaging early social environments.
- We can learn unhelpful behaviour patterns from our care-givers through social learning processes.
- Belief patterns developed in early childhood can lead many individuals to search for negative meanings about themselves in their environments.

5 How is social anxiety kept in place?

In previous chapters I explained what social anxiety is and how it develops. Next, I will look much more specifically at what factors maintain symptoms of social anxiety. Fear of becoming anxious in social situations can lead many of us to invest in different types of protective coping strategies. Being mindful of these coping strategies is important as they can inadvertently maintain symptoms of social anxiety.

The maintenance trio

There are three main ways that most people intuitively react to their social anxiety. These are -

- Worrying about how they will cope in social situations – For example, thinking 'What will it be like tonight...?' The brain will generally send back negative thoughts in response to worry, e.g., "You won't remember people's names"; "You'll feel awkward and uncomfortable"; "You'll come across as boring and uninteresting and people won't want to talk to you."
- Threat monitoring – In social situations this can include continuously monitoring the body for signs of social anxiety, such as feeling awkward, stumbling across words, blushing, etc.

- Behavioural avoidance and safety behaviours – For example, avoiding social situations that may be associated with anxiety, running through mental escape routes, sitting near an exit to keep cool etc.

A further problem tends to occur if the above strategies have been used on a regular basis for a prolonged period of time. If this has been the case for you then it is understandable that it may take may take more time for you to work your way back from experiencing social anxiety symptoms as you will first need to work on breaking habitual patterns associated with the maintenance trio. This may involve deconstructing years of subtle avoidance mechanisms and safety behaviours. (In later chapters we will discuss how you can achieve this). The following chapters will focus on breaking down individual elements of each part of this trio.

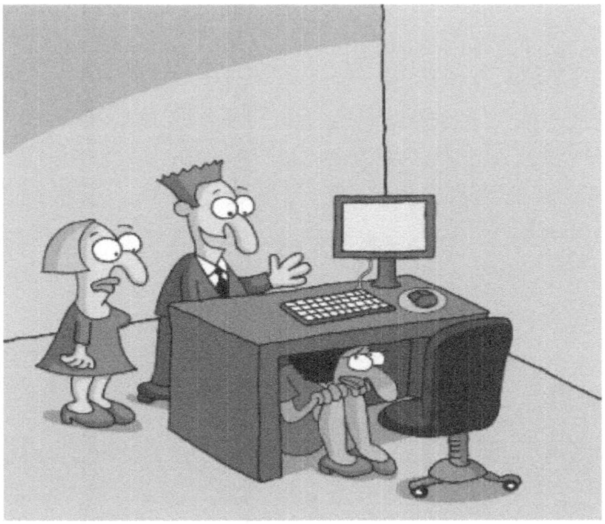

How social anxiety maintains itself

When we carry out certain behaviours and patterns of thinking that we think will help us feel less anxious in social situations we often end up feeling more anxious. Sadly, it is these very behaviours (often referred to as safety behaviours) and thinking patterns that keep our anxiety going and frequently make it worse.

Chapter summary

How is social anxiety kept in place?

- Intuitively doing things to help yourself with symptoms of social anxiety can sometimes make problems worse in the long-term.

- There are three main ways that people react to symptoms of social anxiety. These are a) creating negative thoughts through worry, b) threat monitoring and c) safety behaviours.

6 Worry and social anxiety?

The words *why, what, and how* are engrained in our human psyche. From infancy each of us has an inner tendency to look to understand why the world operates around us the way it does. History informs us that when humans cannot explain why unexplainable processes occur they tend to make hypotheses, or to fill gaps in knowledge using their imagination. In the 15th Century unknown processes may have been referred to as magic, and people of that time may have indulged in superstitious behaviours to protect themselves from things that they didn't understand.

Evolutionary theorists would undoubtedly suggest that our meaning systems are directly linked to our survival, suggesting that our ability to interpret our environment and to make predictions is one factor that has helped humans survive with their comparatively frail mammalian bodies. Indeed, some evolutionary theorists may take this still further stating that it is our human vulnerability itself which has forced our higher cognitive functions to develop more rapidly, leading to humans becoming the most dominant and, arguably, the most dangerous mammal on the surface of the Earth.

> Interestingly, when we know or we 'think' we know we tend to relax a little, even when what we know isn't good news! States of not knowing or perceived uncertainty are highly stressful for creatures that have a natural tendency to search for meaning!

When our search for meaning can make us feel more anxious

A problem can occur when we use higher brain functions to search for answers to an experience of social anxiety that we don't fully understand. Generally, if asked a question the mind will feel compelled to answer and will often trawl through its database before throwing a variety of suggestions into conscious awareness. Typical questions in relation to upcoming social situations often begin with the words "What if?" for example,

"What if I feel awkward tonight?"

"What will it be like tonight?"

"What if my mind goes blank?"

"What if I blush?"

"What if nobody wants to talk to me?"

The mind faced with these types of questions is unlikely to offer up memories about times when you coped well in social situations. Instead, it is more likely to offer thoughts such as "It will be terrible", "It will be really painful." Within this process the mind has the ability to offer information in many different formats, from meaning-based thoughts, to highly vivid images of past events, or potential future events or situations.

Often frightening thoughts (e.g., an image of oneself feeling awkward and embarrassed) are accompanied by high levels of emotional distress as the amygdala in response to fear-based thoughts increases the body's threat response still further. Thus the body can start to produce anxiety symptoms well before social events even occur.

Thoughts and reactions to thoughts that increase the likelihood of feared thoughts occurring

The brains sub-cortical region increases physiological activity in response to threatening ideas generated by higher cortical regions (e.g., "I'm going to blush and everybody is going to notice"). This increase in physiological activity for example, heart rate increase and feeling hot can then be used as evidence for the original thought "I'm going to blush and everybody is going to notice."

This type of pattern is explained nicely using a CBT cycle commonly referred to as a 'Hot Cross Bun,' originally developed by a Psychologist called Christine Padesky, (see figure 6 on the next page).

In this cycle the thought "I am going to blush and everyone is going to notice" results in increased focus on the self. Ultimately, a vicious cycle develops that directly and negatively impacts on the individual concerned.

Figure 6. Maintenance cycle based on Christine Padesky's 'Hot-Cross Bun' approach

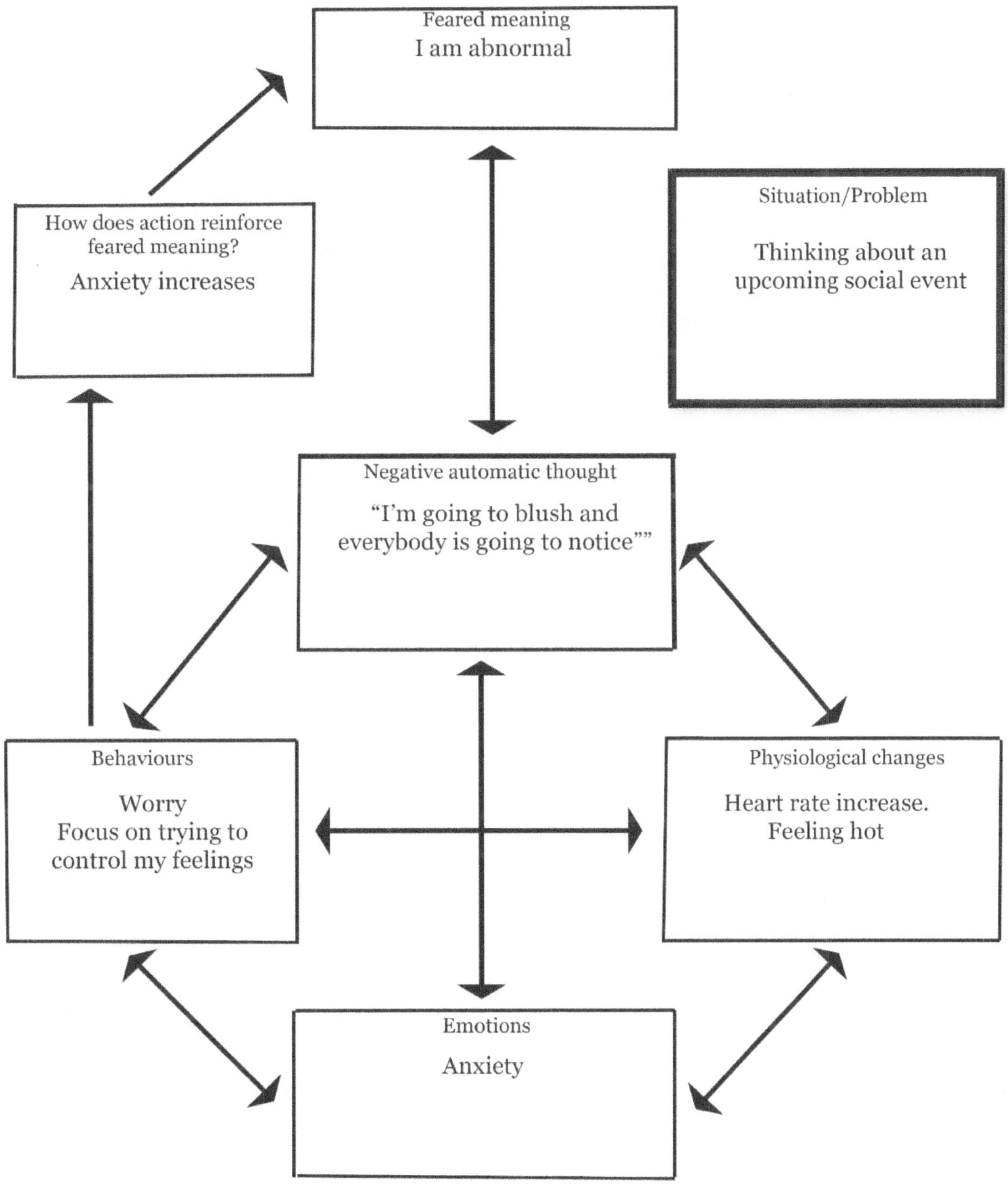

Chapter summary

Worry and social anxiety

- The questions that we ask ourselves can encourage the brain to access frightening thoughts and images.
- Frightening thoughts and images are noticed by the threat perception centre which leads to increased physiological arousal.
- Increased physiological arousal is used as evidence to support the idea that upcoming social events are a threat.

7 Increased threat monitoring and social anxiety

Jenny, a fair haired, university lecturer in her early thirty's, sat in front of me for an initial assessment. A highly intelligent woman with a doctorate in physics, it appeared as though she could barely move in her chair. I asked her what had brought her to therapy, yet it seemed that my questions were deeply painful for her. She was unable to offer any reply apart from "I'm not sure" or "I don't know". She appeared deeply embarrassed by her inability to respond more fully to my questions. More than a minute at a time would pass before Jenny offered even the most simple of responses.

My thinking at the time was that Jenny's threat perception centre had been activated, possibly as a result of being in the presence of an authority type figure (i.e., me), sitting in front of her asking questions. (In line with this I thought that anxiety had temporarily impaired her pre-frontal cortex.) I guessed that Jenny was carrying out a process of self-monitoring, assessing everything that she that she might say and how it might sound. Possibly anything that came to her mind felt like a risk and in this respect she could reduce the risk if she said as little as possible. To test out this idea I moved my chair next to hers, so that she did not feel that she was being directly observed. (This is a common approach that I use in the early stages of therapy with individuals with heightened social anxiety.) Following this, Jenny's anxiety appeared to reduce and she was able to talk much more freely than before. We were then able to complete her assessment.

As our sessions progressed, Jenny and I were able to understand how her threat response was activated based on her past experiences. Jenny had gone to quite extreme lengths to hide her symptoms from others. Her predominant pattern was avoidance. Although her University Department regularly offered social events she managed to avoid all of them, by offering a variety of plausible excuses. Jenny was meticulous with her job, putting in lots of extra time to produce work of a very high standard and she was highly appreciated by her university colleagues.

A particular problem for Jenny was delivering lectures in which she was observed by academics from other universities. This part of her job had become unavoidable. Although Jenny had been able to offer fewer of these types of lectures, the thought of presenting them filled her with dread for weeks or months in advance. Jenny spent enormous amounts of time preparing for her lectures, and rehearsing possible question and answer scenarios. In fact, she reported that her stress levels were so high that on some occasions she had been ready to hand in her resignation but then later changed her mind.

Jenny reported that when faced with unavoidable social situations she had developed a number of coping strategies. Jenny had a fear of her mind going blank when she was anxious and didn't trust what she might say in these situations. As a result of this she would spend time repeating what she wanted to say over and over in her mind before saying anything. On some occasions she repeated what she was going to say in her mind so many times that she forgot what was being discussed. This led to her feeling highly embarrassed, (see figure 5). I will explain why this process occurs in later chapters.

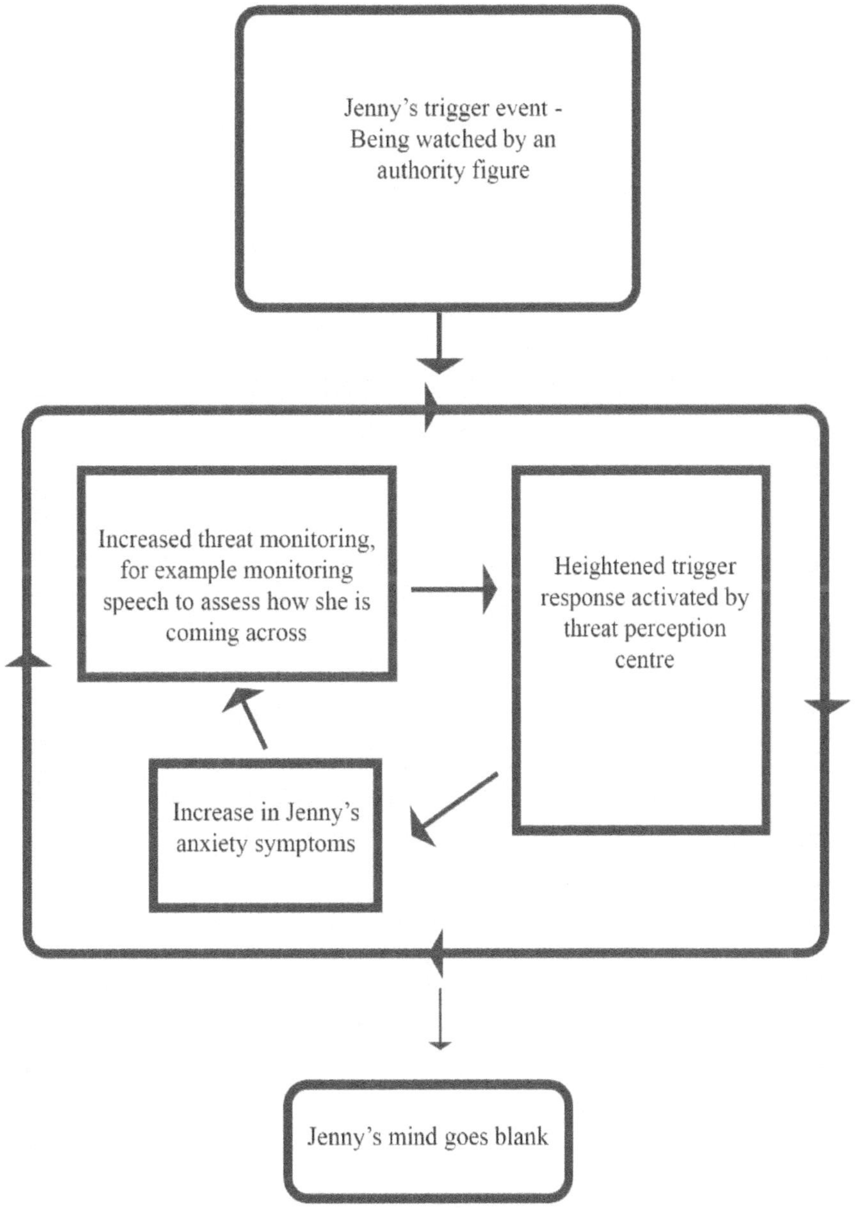

Figure 7. Impact of threat monitoring on Jenny's symptoms of social anxiety.

Chapter summary

Increased threat monitoring and social anxiety

- The threat perception system naturally screens for symptoms of anxiety, especially if social events have been perceived as psychologically threatening in the past.
- Focusing on changes in the body and viewing body changes as a threat increases the intensity of anxiety sensations.
- Regularly screening the body increases sensitivity to feelings and reinforces to the sub-cortical mind that bodily changes are indeed a genuine threat!

8 Behavioural avoidance and safety behaviours

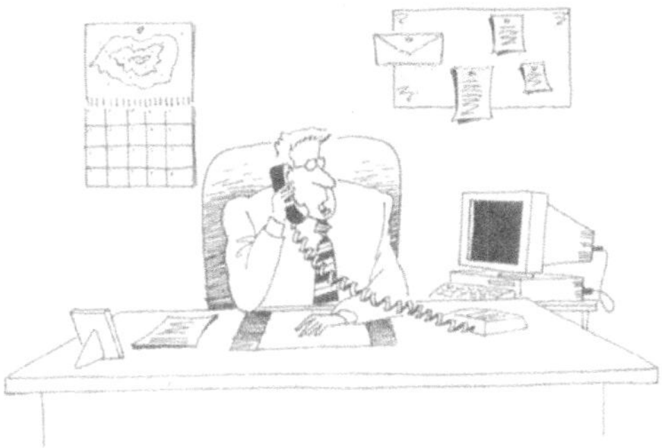

"Oh, just thinking of ways to avoid everyone I work with. And you?"

Gregory M. was an energetic 26-year-old young father of two small children. He was an international I.T. expert and regularly travelled the world to head up think tanks, to offer formal presentations, and to help different teams work together more effectively. He was very highly thought of by his employers and had recently been promoted to Vice President by his US-based company. Along with his wife, and his General Practitioner I was one of the few people to whom he had disclosed his difficulties.

Gregory's main focus was concealing any sense of vulnerability. Gregory told me that he felt panicky in many different types of situations but did everything he could to hide it. In his mind Gregory expected himself to appear confident, in control, able, articulate, sociable, and intelligent at all times. In many respects Gregory described his life much like an acting performance that he needed to deliver perfectly day after day. When offering presentations he tended to worry about his voice trembling and worried about his heart rate rising. To cope with these problems Gregory took a beta-blocker before making formal presentations. To help him with concerns about his voice he recruited a voice expert to strengthen it. He had a developed an array of very sophisticated and rehearsed avoidance mechanisms that he used if he noticed himself becoming anxious during a presentation. He had physical props in place that he could utilise or he had excuses pre-planned which would give him an opportunity to leave the room for a few minutes. He had learnt how to do all of these things while coming across completely naturally.

Around his friends Gregory painted a picture of himself as a confident person, again using a set of tools designed to avoid showing any type of vulnerability. Gregory limited his alcohol intake during social occasions for fear of saying or doing something stupid. He didn't disclose any of his life difficulties even to his best friends. Gregory said that on reflection the only person that he shared his insecurities with was his wife, and that even his best friend didn't really know him.

A particular problem for Gregory was that recently he had started to become much more avoidant about chairing meetings in person and had started offering conference calls instead. Nobody at his company had said anything about this to him, although it was a particular source of concern for him as being physically present with people was fundamental to his work role.

After meeting Gregory my initial opinion was that he was quite a long way down the social anxiety path as he had several avoidant behaviours and safety mechanisms already in place. It seemed as though he was stuck in an acting role that he did not know how to extricate himself from. He had become tired and fatigued as a result of his constant need to perform. I thought that he needed to become more aware of many of his many subtle avoidance strategies and safety behaviours before he could address the root cause of his problem which was his fear that deep down inside there was something intrinsically wrong with him.

The type of avoidance and safety behaviours demonstrated by Gregory are quite common. Many sufferers keep their problems a secret. In fact, Gregory had hidden his symptoms so well that it would have been a big surprise to others to discover just how socially anxious he really was.

Becoming an expert in social avoidance

As time progresses many individuals with social anxiety develop a number of imaginative strategies to control or avoid feeling anxious in social situations. Many are skilled in dealing with social anxiety, having becoming experts in developing strategies to avoid it or neutralise it. This behaviour is not surprising, not only due to an inclination to avoid high levels of anxiety, but also because it's natural to want to avoid potentially harmful social outcomes.

Conditioned responses

There is a major problem with using avoidance and safety behaviours to reduce social anxiety, however. The more that we carry out safety behaviours the more engrained these behaviours become. We are preprogramed to experience a sense of relief (which acts as negative reinforcement) when we engage in a behaviour that removes pain or reduces worry (see figures 8) Over time as this process is repeated, memory pathways are laid down and we may begin to carry out these behaviours automatically outside of conscious awareness.

Initially, to Gregory's it appeared that the more avoidant strategies and safety behaviours he used the less anxiety others noticed in him. In this respect, in the early stages he may have felt as though he was dealing successfully with his problem. As time progressed however, he started to feel more anxious than he did previously (see figure 9).

What is negative reinforcement?

Negative reinforcement occurs when something is removed or taken away (often pain or anxiety) as a result of a particular behaviour. For example, for some people making a decision that they do not need to travel on a plane or a tube can take away their anxiety giving them an immediate sense of relief. Generally, the more an individual uses a behaviour (e.g., taking a pain killer) to remove a stimulus (e.g., pain) the more automatic the behaviour becomes.

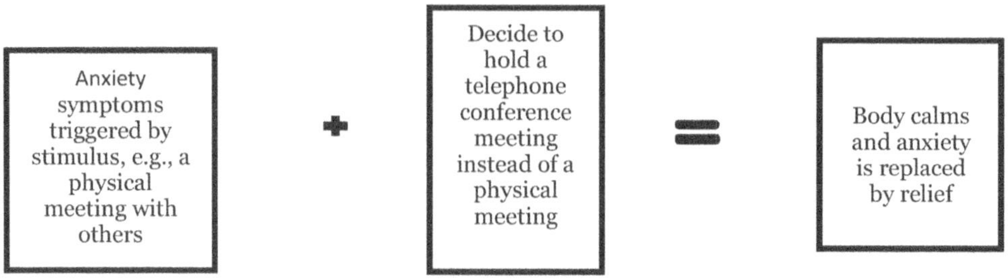

Figure 8. How negative reinforcement develops during a process of avoidance.

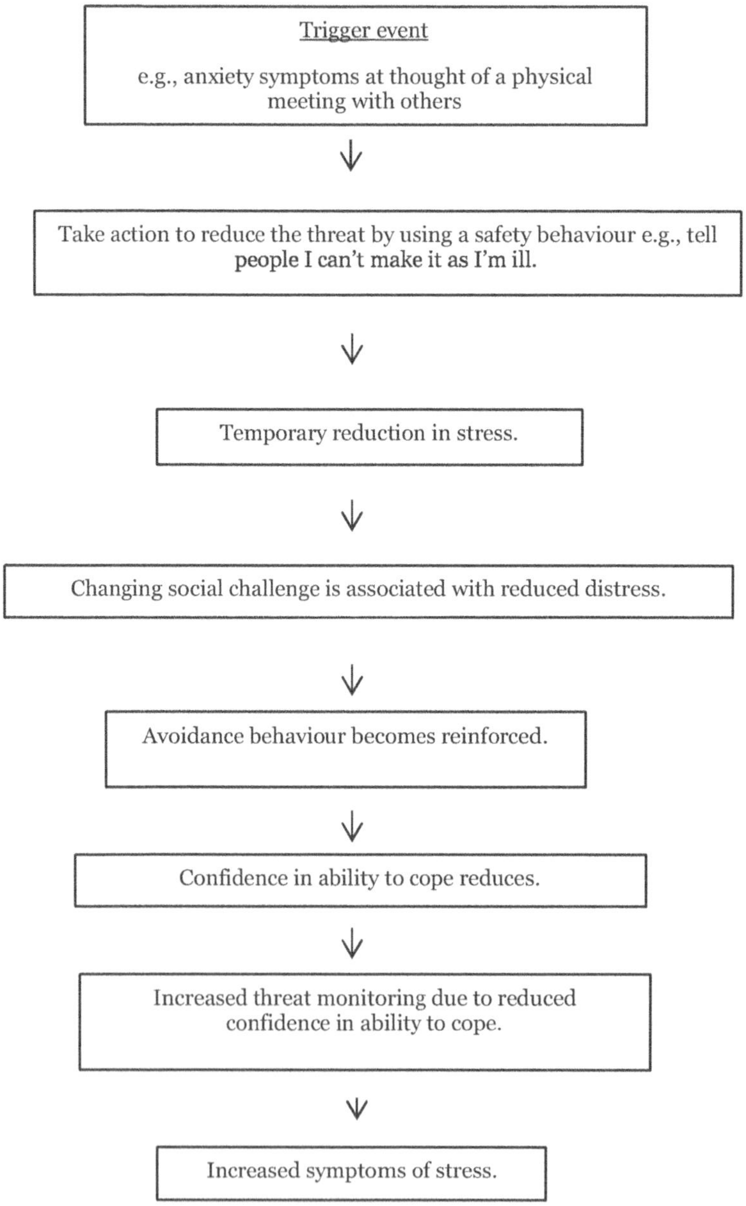

Figure 9. Impact of avoidance and safety behaviours on symptoms of anxiety.

Chapter summary

Behavioural avoidance and safety behaviours

- Our natural inclination is to move away from or avoid pain (e.g., anxiety).
- Through a process of trial and error we find out what behaviours result in our anxiety reducing (e.g., distraction, avoidance etc.).
- A process of negative reinforcement occurs as our brains make a connection between the use of safety behaviours and feeling relieved.
- Safety behaviours become engrained and automatic over time.
- Our lives become more restricted and our confidence in coping with social events reduces.

Chapter 8 – Homework

If you want to, you can use the table on the next page to make a note of the safety behaviours that you use to protect yourself in social environments (see table 1 overleaf). Using table 2, keep a record about how much you believe that this behaviour has stopped something dangerous happening to you or kept you safe. Rate your belief between 0 and 10, where 10 means that you totally believe it.

Table 2. Safety behaviour record

Use this diary to make a note of safety behaviours you use each time you feel socially anxious. Keep a record also about how much you believe that this behaviour has stopped something happening or kept you safe. Rate your belief between 0 and 10 where 10 means that you totally believe it.

Date/Time	Social situation	Safety behaviour, e.g., Go somewhere with a safe person.	Anxiety rating after safety behaviour	How much do you believe your safety behaviour protected you from something happening? Score out of 10.
8pm 12th August	At theatre	While in the foyer focussed on myself to make sure that I was coming across normally	6	7

Table 1. Safety behaviours when socially anxious **(Use the box to the right to note which safety behaviours apply to you)**	✓
Use diazepam or beta-blockers before social events e.g., business meetings.	
Carry a supply of diazepam just in case.	
Drink alcohol before going out to relax.	
Avoid situations where social anxiety has occurred in the past or where it may occur in the future.	
Go to the toilet before going out (related to fear of using lavatories and others over-hearing)	
Have someone safe with you when going to social situations.	
Carry a bottle of water (to help with a dry mouth).	
Sit close to an exit so as to escape unnoticed.	
Hold onto or lean onto something supportive to hide shaking or trembling.	
Wear light clothing, fan self or stand near a window or a doorway to prevent over-heating.	
Wear extra clothes to conceal sweating.	
Have tissue ready to wipe hands to conceal sweaty hands.	
Use heavy makeup to avoid others noticing blushing or cover face with hair.	
Drink out a bottle rather than a glass to avoid others noticing shaking hands.	
Have stories ready to put on an act of social competence and to have something interesting to say.	
Focus on self to assess social performance.	
Avoid conversations with people.	
Stand in a corner to keep a low profile.	
Keep conversations as short as possible to avoid revealing anything that could be self-incriminating.	
Focus on appearance.	
Try to control facial expressions.	
Avoid eye-contact with others.	
Mentally rehearse what is being said before it is said.	
Have excuses about a need to leave pre-planned and ready.	
Keep asking questions so as to appear interested.	
Total number of safety behaviours endorsed.	

Table 2. Safety behaviour record

Use this diary to make a note of safety behaviours you use each time you feel socially anxious. Keep a record also about how much you believe that this behaviour has stopped something happening or kept you safe. Rate your belief between 0 and 10 where 10 means that you totally believe it.				
Date/Time	**Social situation**	**Safety behaviour, e.g., Go somewhere with a safe person.**	**Anxiety rating after safety behaviour**	**How much do you believe your safety behaviour protected you from something happening? Score out of 10.**

Table 2. Safety behaviour record

Use this diary to make a note of safety behaviours you use each time you feel socially anxious. Keep a record also about how much you believe that this behaviour has stopped something happening or kept you safe. Rate your belief between 0 and 10 where 10 means that you totally believe it.

Date/Time	**Social situation**	**Safety behaviour, e.g., Go somewhere with a safe person.**	**Anxiety rating after safety behaviour**	**How much do you believe your safety behaviour protected you from something happening? Score out of 10.**

9

Connecting the dots

A good deal of information has been covered up to this point. With this in mind, it will be useful to reflect on what has been covered so far before progressing any further.

In chapter one I described how disabling social anxiety can be, and how social anxiety can arise as a result of both genetic factors and the environments that people are brought up in. I also suggested that a problem that many individuals with social anxiety face is that painful childhood interpersonal experiences can become stored within the sub-cortical brain's memory system, which I called the threat perception centre (see chapter 3).

The threat perception centre in completing its function effectively, screens the individual's internal and external environment for cues that are connected to past traumatic experiences. If trauma cues, negative beliefs, or negative assumptions are detected the threat perception centre will trigger an anxiety response to help the individual prepare for the threat. Following this, the individual is more likely to do two things at the same time 1) focus on the threat and 2) attempt to get rid of the threat, often by using safety behaviours. Continuous attempts to get rid of a threat by using safety behaviours can lead to these behaviours becoming more automatic as a result of negative reinforcement (see figure 10).

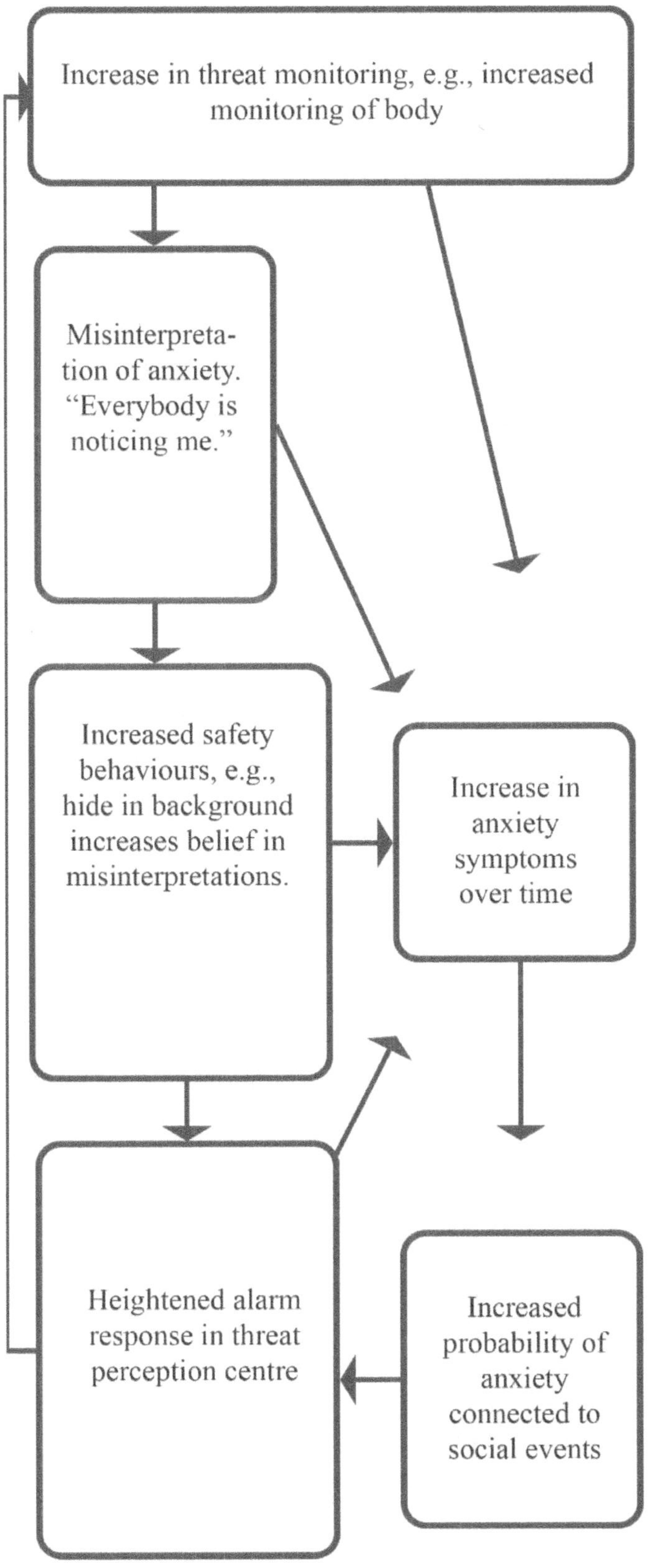

Figure 10. Maintenance cycle of social anxiety

I mentioned earlier that professors Clarke and Wells' thought a lot about this area in the early 1990's, before they developed their 1995 model of social anxiety. Their model suggested that social anxiety starts with a triggering situation that can activate an individual's beliefs and assumptions. As a result of **beliefs** - fears about the self which we believe to be true - becoming activated the body produces an anxiety response and the individuals carry out safety behaviours in an attempt to get rid of, or conceal, symptoms of anxiety. While carrying out safety behaviours individuals become focused on the self and pre-occupied with signs and symptoms of anxiety, which generally leads to increased symptoms of anxiety. Individuals then use their struggle to cope with the aforementioned situation as further evidence for their beliefs and assumptions.

I will explain how this model works by looking at problems experienced by Alice J. Alice J feels anxious in response to noticing her cheeks becoming warm. Alice, who holds a belief that she is abnormal carries out a safety behaviour of fanning herself to cool down to prevent her face becoming red (see figure 11). This process encourages her to focus more on herself as she monitors the heat in her face. The process of monitoring the heat in her face triggers further anxiety and she feels her face beginning to heat up. Alice leaves the room to go and splash water on her face to cool herself down. This whole process is used by Alice as confirmatory

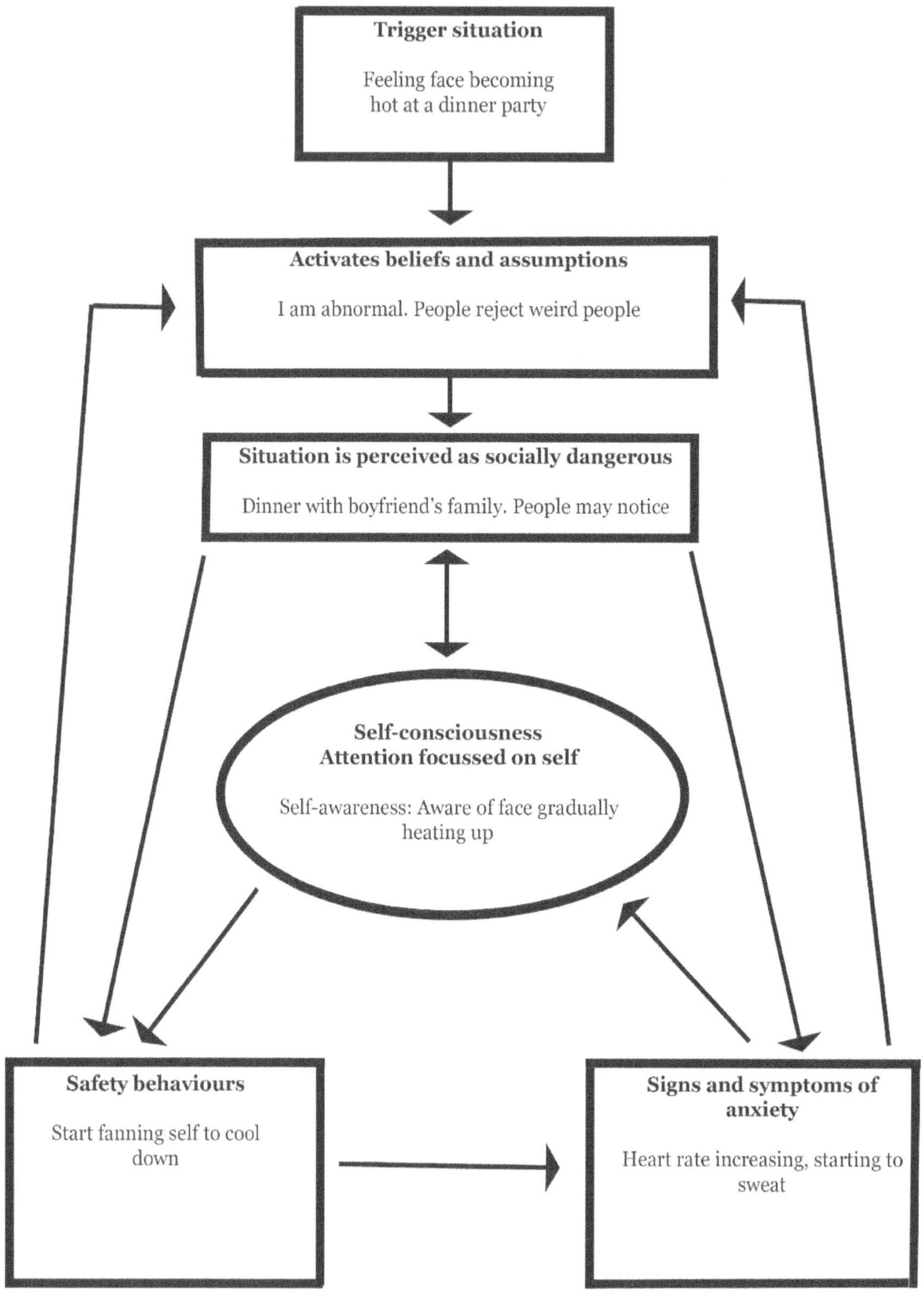

Figure 11. Example of Clark and Wells maintenance model of anxiety (1995)

evidence that a) social situations are a threat and b) her beliefs and assumptions are accurate, e.g., I am abnormal. Nobody else fans themselves or needs to leave the room to cool down.

In common with most CBT models Clarke and Wells' model describes a self-fulfilling prophesy. Ultimately, their suggestion is that safety behaviours used to disguise symptoms of anxiety end up reinforcing the individuals' worst fears, e.g., I am abnormal.

Examples of social anxiety leading to self-fulfilling prophesies are quite common. For example, if we look at Jenny the Physicist. With unknown people - but especially authority figures – When she is asked a question Jenny rehearses in her mind what she is going to say before she speaks. This problem becomes exacerbated when she is anxious. While thinking about what she wants to say Jenny forgets what the question is and needs to ask what the question is again. To others who are not aware of what is going on in Jenny's mind, they are left to draw their own conclusions. Some people may recognise that Jenny feels anxious, some may think that the question stimulated a creative thinking process which distracted her, others may think that she was not interested in the question. Jenny feels that others think that she is stupid and berates herself. The cycle continues.

Other examples of self-fulfilling prophecies

Jane fears being disliked by others. As a safety behaviour she declines social invitations or often cancels at the last minute. Over time, social invitations dry up as people think that Jane is not interested in their invitations or they expect Jane to decline. Jane becomes upset when she discovers that some of her friends have been invited to another friend's party and she hasn't.

At an event with people he hasn't met before Joseph worries about coming across as boring and being rejected. To protect himself from his fear he is careful about what he says and speaks very little. People talk much more to each other than Joseph. People find out very little about Joseph which gives them less opportunity to initiate future conversations with him. As time progresses Joseph notices other people in the group having interesting conversations with each other and forming friendships. Joseph does not feel included in the group and wonders why new groups don't appear to accept him.

John is concerned about coming across as odd or weird. He is highly anxious and in social interactions he focusses on himself to assess how he may appear to others. As a result, John does not have the attentional capacity to listen to what others are saying to him at the same time. John's conversations are very disjointed. Others who interact with him start to feel awkward and struggle with the effort of maintaining conversation with him. They gradually find others to talk to. The whole process reinforces to John how weird and odd he is.

Chapter summary
Connecting the dots

- Clarke and Wells' (1995) model of social anxiety suggests that anxiety starts with a triggering situation that activates beliefs and assumptions.
- Clarke and Wells' model of social anxiety suggests that behaviours that individuals carry out to protect themselves from what they fear create a self-fulfilling prophesy.
- Safety behaviours carried out to conceal anxiety reinforce individuals' fears and beliefs, thereby maintaining their problems.

10 Some key terms

Luckily there are several different ways to intervene with social anxiety symptoms. They can be challenged by a) understanding much more about how social anxiety works, b) behavioural interventions, c) cognitive interventions and d) using a combined cognitive and behavioural approach. I would like to define these key concepts for you now, so that you become familiar with them.

Behavioural strategies

Behavioural strategies are often used in working with social anxiety. This might mean making a small adjustment to what you do or altering your environment in some way. Often, the use of behavioural strategies can bring anxiety levels down sufficiently so that other cognitive strategies work more successfully.

Cognitive strategies or interventions

Cognitive interventions are essentially strategies that you can use mainly within your mind. In particular, cognitive interventions require you to react differently to your thoughts and feelings. Cognitive strategies tend to work more successfully when anxiety levels are lower. This is because (as I mentioned earlier) the neocortex (which is used more so for cognitive approaches) tends to go off-line (has reduced capacity/capability) at times of heightened anxiety.

Cognitive behaviour therapy

To make permanent changes to your symptoms of social anxiety you will eventually use a combined cognitive and behavioural approach. This will involve using your new cognitive and behavioural tools while you approach previously feared situations. You will read about this later when I present you with an opportunity to reprogram your sub-cortical mind, or at least help it become less active in situations that currently produce high levels of fear.

Chapter summary

Some key terms

- Behavioural strategies will require you to make changes to your behaviour and to measure the impact of those changes.
- Cognitive strategies are interventions that you use with your mind.
- Cognitive behavioural strategies are a combination of both the above.

11

It may feel real but does that make it real?

A process of changing old ways of thinking and behaving in social environments is likely to cause you uncertainty at both a logical and a feeling level. I have found that it is slightly easier to accomplish behaviour change, if the logic behind behaviour change is explained very clearly. I have therefore written this chapter to offer you some factual information about social anxiety.

What impact does self-focussed thinking have on cognitive processes?

Earlier, I described the presenting problems experienced by Jenny the Physicist. Jenny's most dominant safety behaviour was to monitor what she was going to say before she spoke. In order to accomplish her safety behaviour Jenny needed to use a part of her brain devoted to **working memory**. Working memory is a cognitive process that we use to hold information in our mind and to manipulate it at the same time. We use working memory for mental arithmetic (i.e., doing sums without a calculator) or to remember a telephone number that someone has just shouted to us across a room. A number of scientific studies have shown that working memory capacity is limited to an average of between five and nine units of information. Research from several scientific studies also shows that working memory capacity reduces still further when we become anxious.

When Jenny rehearses what she says before she says it, she is using up working memory capacity. When Jenny forgets a question it is because there isn't sufficient room to hold the question and her rehearsed answer in her working memory at the same time. This doesn't make Jenny stupid, it simply means that her working memory capacity has reached its limit. The same problem would occur for any of us no matter how intelligent we are. Self-monitoring also uses up working memory capacity. In this respect, if you are screening yourself - your internal environment - for symptoms of anxiety then you will find it extremely difficult to focus on your external environment at the same time. Thus, it will be very difficult for you to truly attend to what others are saying. As a result of this, self-monitoring can lead to disjointed and awkward conversations. It can also lead to difficulties keeping up with conversations, and it can create problems following instructions offered by others.

In a state of anxiety our thinking patterns change and we do not process information accurately

As I mentioned earlier when the threat perception centre activates the body's natural alarm system the body moves into a state of preparation. This can have an obvious impact on the body's biological system, but significantly, it can also alter the way that the brain processes information.

Cognitive distortions were originally described by Aaron Beck, a founder of modern CBT, in his 1976 book "Cognitive Therapies and Emotional Disorders". I have placed a list of cognitive distortions on the next page, see table 3. When we enter a state of high emotional arousal we engage automatically in more primitive thinking and perceive the world in a distorted way.

Table 3. Cognitive distortions

Thinking biases and what to look out for

All or nothing thinking: Viewing things as either right or wrong; there is no middle ground. Things are either perfect or fundamentally flawed. There is just black or white, grey does not exist, e.g., always/never, good/bad.

Personalising: Focussing on things in the immediate environment and connecting it to the self. Thinking for example, "she did that deliberately because she knew that I wouldn't like that!" The world revolves around the self.

Mental filtering: Selecting specific negative ideas to dwell on and ignoring all of the positive ones.

Disqualifying the positive: Positives don't count, there is nothing special about the way I did it, e.g., "That only happened because I was lucky."

Distorted images: Using images as evidence. A picture or image in the mind that reflects extreme themes of fear, sadness, disgust, pain, etc.

Fortune telling: Predicting the future in a negative way without any real evidence, e.g., "It's going to be terrible", "It will be a disaster", "I just know it."

Shoulds, oughts & musts: Having ideas that things can only be done one way: - "People should ...", "I must ...", "I really ought to ...", "He shouldn't have ..."

Over-generalising: Taking single events or circumstances and viewing them as happening more often than they really do. Thinking that things happen everywhere.

Emotional reasoning: Using emotions as evidence, e.g., "I feel it, so it must be true."

Mind reading: Drawing conclusions about what others are thinking without any evidence, e.g., "She doesn't like me", They think I am stupid."

As you may imagine with cognitive distortions becoming active when you are anxious it is very unlikely that you will see a realistic or accurate version of events within your social environment.

Generally, most non-socially anxious people are unaware of minor symptoms of anxiety such as shaking or blushing, or are simply not bothered by it. Realistically, the people who are most likely to notice these types of symptoms are individuals with social anxiety who often compare themselves with others. Bear in mind, however, that these individuals will be far too busy self-monitoring and focussing on themselves to be looking at you.

What is normal when faced with a new social situation?

Most people when faced with a novel social situation will experience some anxiety. Many people with social anxiety have concerns about being judged and believe that if they come across as confident and socially skilled then people will like them. In fact, there is no evidence that this is the case. People who are socially skilled may well attend more social events, however, they can be equally loved and disliked by others.

How do I develop social skills?

There are no specific rules for social skills, although formalities can be observed for different types of situations. Generally, the environment will dictate what kind of formalities are in operation and as such rules can easily be garnered by watching others, for example, noticing what clothes others wear, or what order they do things in. It seems that most of us develop social skills naturally and more effectively by not focussing on developing skills. I can state with certainty that focusing on your social skills while you interact with others is likely to disrupt the natural flow of your communication and reduce your emotional connection with others.

When trying to be invisible gets you noticed more

A common coping strategy that I have come across with some clients is an attempt to project an air of invisibility to help reduce anxiety. They may focus on themselves to assess how they are coming across to others. They may try to avoid eye contact because they think it will make themselves or others feel uncomfortable. They may attempt to avoid sharing anything personal, even though others may be interested in finding out more about them. Some may cancel social invites at the last minute or avoid social situations altogether to protect themselves from being judged by others. All of the above attempts at invisibility can lead to you drawing more attention to yourself. For example, if I were your host I would notice or be disappointed if you cancelled, and I would be aware if you left without saying goodbye.

It

Chapter summary

It may feel real but does that make it real?

- Self-focussed thinking and self-monitoring uses up working memory capacity. If you do this you will not be able to concentrate effectively in social environments.

- In a state of heightened emotional arousal thinking patterns come on line which distort perception. When we are anxious we do not view our environment or events accurately.

- Feeling anxious is normal and you will not improve your social skills by focusing on your social skills.

- Trying to be invisible may end up with you drawing more attention to yourself.

12 Creating your own hypotheses

A **hypothesis** is a prediction about what you think will occur based on what you think you know. Most of us create hypotheses all of the time in our daily interactions with others. We make hypotheses when we think about how others may think or behave in response to what we do. For example, when I'm in my car queuing in traffic and I want to move into the next lane I know that if I put my indicator on and start edging out slightly, eventually there will be someone who is generous enough in spirit to let me move in front of them.

In my work with clients I also follow a hypothesis driven approach. By this I mean I continuously make educated guesses about what is troubling someone using the information that they have given me. Equally, I actively encourage my clients to engage in a process of making predictions about how they might think, feel, and behave in various situations. In the chapters that follow, you will be offered a chance to test several things out, to create new psychological explanations – or psychological formulations - that will help you move forward in managing your social anxiety.

After you understand what is happening to you, you will then be better placed to try out new coping strategies while you are in situations that make you feel anxious. An idea behind carrying out new strategies is to help you find out if making little changes here and there produces different results. I can't stress how important it is that you give yourself the opportunity to try alternative strategies to assess what impact they have on the way you feel. When this occurs you will be able to a) learn from your new experiences and b) repeat similar processes in the future, hopefully even for the rest of your life. Expect resistance from yourself when you complete CBT. Recognise also that if you can pass through this resistance you may learn new things from your experiences. You can also use what you learn in the future, hopefully even for the rest of your life.

To illustrate this I'd like you to imagine there's a fictional reader of this book called Tom Pooley. Let's say that Tom has been social anxious for several years and he has now picked up this book and is reading it. Based on the information offered, Tom creates a hypothesis that many different areas of his life have had an impact on his experience of social anxiety. After reading further in this book he makes a predication that if he reacts to his feelings in a different way his anxiety is likely to reduce. Once Tom has this prediction in place (i.e., his new hypothesis) he is reluctant to test it out as it is unfamiliar to him. Eventually, however, he allows himself to get curious enough about what may occur if he behaves differently. After Tom has tested out this new idea he **reflects** – which means that he thinks about the changes that he has noticed. This process of reflection helps Tom to firm up his new approach in his mind which in turn encourages him to repeat similar approaches later on.

Fear of change

In my twenty or so years as a psychologist fear of change has cropped up frequently in my professional life. Embarrassingly, I will admit to you now that I initially resist learning new therapeutic approaches thinking my current approach is the best way. I then approach the new therapy area and feel fear, anxiety, and uncertainty while I learn to practice it. At this point these new approaches represent a challenge to my previous view of what I thought I knew and I feel generally incompetent. I then gain the necessary knowledge about using the new approach and my confidence in using it increases. The process then starts over again. Each time I do this I learn new things to extend my knowledge and understanding.

Although CBT is logical and scientific, carrying out CBT approaches will be a challenge to you. Changes in thinking do not happen that readily. Even when change is regarded as good, our natural human tendency is to put up resistance. When you experience this resistance, recognise that your resistance is part of a process of learning. Use it to take you forward. When you take yourself forward your learning will become **experiential** as well as logical. Experiential learning means learning by doing, rather than learning about something by reading or thinking about it.

Chapter summary

Creating your own hypotheses

- We use hypotheses to make predictions about what we think will occur based on the knowledge we have.
- We tend to fear change and put up resistance when we are faced with doing something we don't fully understand.
- A process of significant change moves through a predetermined order – Uncertainty, experiential learning, and then reflection, which in turn leads to a new level of certainty.

13 Observe yourself

In many respects it could be suggested that learning how to think about your thinking is a corner stone of CBT. In this vein of thought, to get the most out of your CBT you will need to operate a little bit like a scientist, stepping back and becoming aware of a) how you think b) how you relate to your feelings and c) the behavioural choices you make. Thinking scientifically you can then make small changes here and there, assess the impact of these changes, and if necessary, make further small adjustments. Obviously, small changes and adjustments by themselves will not make a significant difference to your life, but it is reasonable to assume that an accumulation of hundreds of them will.

A commonly offered piece of advice in many CBT books is to write a journal to chart your progress. In practice, I have found that many people nod their head, agree that this it is a good idea, but rarely get past the stage of writing a few lines in a note book. This could be because most people do not really understand why it is necessary to keep a record of progress or they may prefer not to write things down for fear of personal information being read by others.

With this in mind, I would like to sell you an idea of writing things down for one major reason. Our working memory capacity is very small. Thinking about your thoughts without writing them down on paper increases the cognitive load that you are placing on your working memory. In contrast, having your thoughts written down in front of you makes them much easier to manipulate and reduces cognitive load.

Keeping a record in a notebook or a computer can also be a very useful memory aid if in the future you wish to remind yourself about what you have learnt. Many of us forget how we made our progress. In fact, although many CBT studies indicate that distress reduces significantly after CBT intervention, they also show quite a strong relapse effect over the passage of time. The practice of noting down your thoughts will therefore give you an opportunity to train your brain to reflect on a regular basis. This process of refection is used frequently by CBT therapists working in clinical practice. Questions such as "What did you make of that?", "What did you learn as a result of trying that?" are commonplace. Therapists engage their clients in this reflective activity to help their clients draw attention to thoughts that may otherwise remain in the background of their minds. You can benefit from this type of process without using a therapist by setting aside some time to carry out this reflective activity on your own.

Completing thought records

In 1995 Dennis Greenberger and Christine Padesky dedicated practically a whole book (Mind Over Mood) to completing thought records. Thoughts records alone will not significantly change your life but they will allow you to choose how to react to the thoughts that lie in the background of your mind influencing the way that you feel. I have placed a section of thought record for you to have a look at on the next page, (see table 4). I have also placed further blank sheets at the end of this chapter. Using these sheets will allow you to keep a permanent record of your experiences.

To complete thought records effectively you will need to begin observing yourself very carefully. The first thing that I will invite you to notice is that you are having thoughts and feelings. The second thing that I would like you to recognise is that you have a range of thoughts, feelings, and behaviours in different circumstances. Once you become aware that your thoughts and feelings fluctuate, you can monitor how you react in different situations.

Ideally, you will approach your thoughts with an intention of becoming really curious about what you will notice. Try to develop an interest in the different types of thoughts that you experience and the feelings or sensations that accompany your thoughts. Carrying out self-observation is not designed to encourage you to judge yourself: Bear in mind that noticing a critical or self-judgemental thought is very different to listening to or believing a thought.

My experience of CBT

When I first had CBT, I had an aversion to writing and filling in charts. Writing things down didn't really appeal to me. I thought that it might work much better for others, but not for me. Eventually, my therapist Jenny convinced me to fill in the sheets and I found that they actually helped with my mood. I noticed I could stand back from myself more. I started to realise I had many more feelings than I previously thought. I saw that a lot of the things

Automatic thoughts, e.g. "She doesn't like me"	Physiology, e.g. chest tightening	Emotion, e.g. anxiety	Behaviour, e.g. avoid contact with that person
"This is terrible. Why does it have to be like this?" "Why does this keep happening?" "I'll be a laughing stock." "I look so incompetent" "Laura is bound to have second thoughts about me." "I'm sure Laura's brother thinks I'm strange"	Hands shaking Legs trembling Feel hot Chest tight Tense in the back of the neck	Anxious Embarrassed	Try to hold onto glass firmly to hide my hands shaking. Focus on myself and say very little.

Table 4. Thoughts, physiology, emotion and behaviour diary

I was doing in my personal life I didn't actually enjoy. I started to see that there were things missing from my life. I wasn't consciously aware of these things before I started observing myself. Once I realised there was a primitive – or feeling - part to the mind, I began to notice when it came on-line much more and how it affected the way that I thought. I recognised that my analytical mind and my feeling mind didn't always agree. I started listening to both parts of my mind and then making decisions after thinking about my life in a more balanced way.

It wasn't obvious to me before I began observing myself that for every thought, feeling, or behaviour I noticed, I had a choice about how to react or respond. Before CBT, I was just living a bit like a puppet, acting automatically. It also helped me not to judge my thoughts and feelings. I felt so much more confident once I noticed I didn't need to react to every thought or feeling that I had.

What information is collected using thought records?

When you record your **physiological reactions** this means looking at specific bodily changes that occur in your body. Specific body changes that you may record could be increased tension, emptiness, a tight chest, a pounding head, your heart racing, heavy feelings in the legs, and such like. The information that you record in the emotions section is the label that you give to specific bodily changes. Many physiological reactions connected to emotions are very similar. For example, the physiological changes associated with anxiety and anger both involve a) heart rate increase, b) a rise on blood pressure, c) tension in major muscle groups, and such like. However, similar bodily reactions can be perceived very differently, and trigger different consequential behaviours.

There are many different variations of self-observation diaries used in CBT, but most involve recording combinations of thoughts, physiological reactions, feelings/emotions, and behaviours. Diaries encourage the use of regular body scanning, which will be beneficial to you as body scanning a) evokes greater sensory awareness and b) encourages increased experiential learning. I mentioned earlier that experiential learning occurs when people learn through their senses and feelings, rather than through thinking or reading.

Following the completion of a thought record you can if you wish take things further by arranging your material into a CBT cycle. The cycle that I use most in clinical practice is an adapted version of the Padesky hot-cross bun which I have drawn for you on the next page. Ostensibly, you will be using the same information that you have in your thoughts, feelings, and behaviour record, but you will be arranging the information slightly differently. The process of arranging material into this cycle is important as it will a) encourage you to recognise the self-defeating cycles that you engage in and b) help you to look at yourself more objectively and less subjectively.

Can self-observation increase the effectiveness of the pre-frontal cortex?

The brain is well-known by **neurologists** - who are medical experts in the brain - to have high levels of **plasticity**. Plasticity means that the brain has the ability to repair itself and grow in size the more that it is used. Neuropsychologist, Professor Eleanor Maguire from Ireland has published over 100 research articles and book chapters on the neuropsychology of the brain. The majority of her research has focussed on memory, the hippocampus (an important brain area connected to memory) and the sub-cortical brain regions surrounding it. In perhaps one of her most famous papers dating back to the 1990's, she and her colleagues reported the results of their investigation into the brains of London taxi drivers. London taxi drivers were a very useful 'real life' experiment at the time, as there was a requirement that all taxi drivers complete a process known as the 'knowledge.' This required London taxi drivers to spend a large amount of time memorising the spatial layout of London streets - or exercising their hippocampi. If they did not pass the 'knowledge' test they could not become a taxi driver in London. Eleanor Maguire used a process

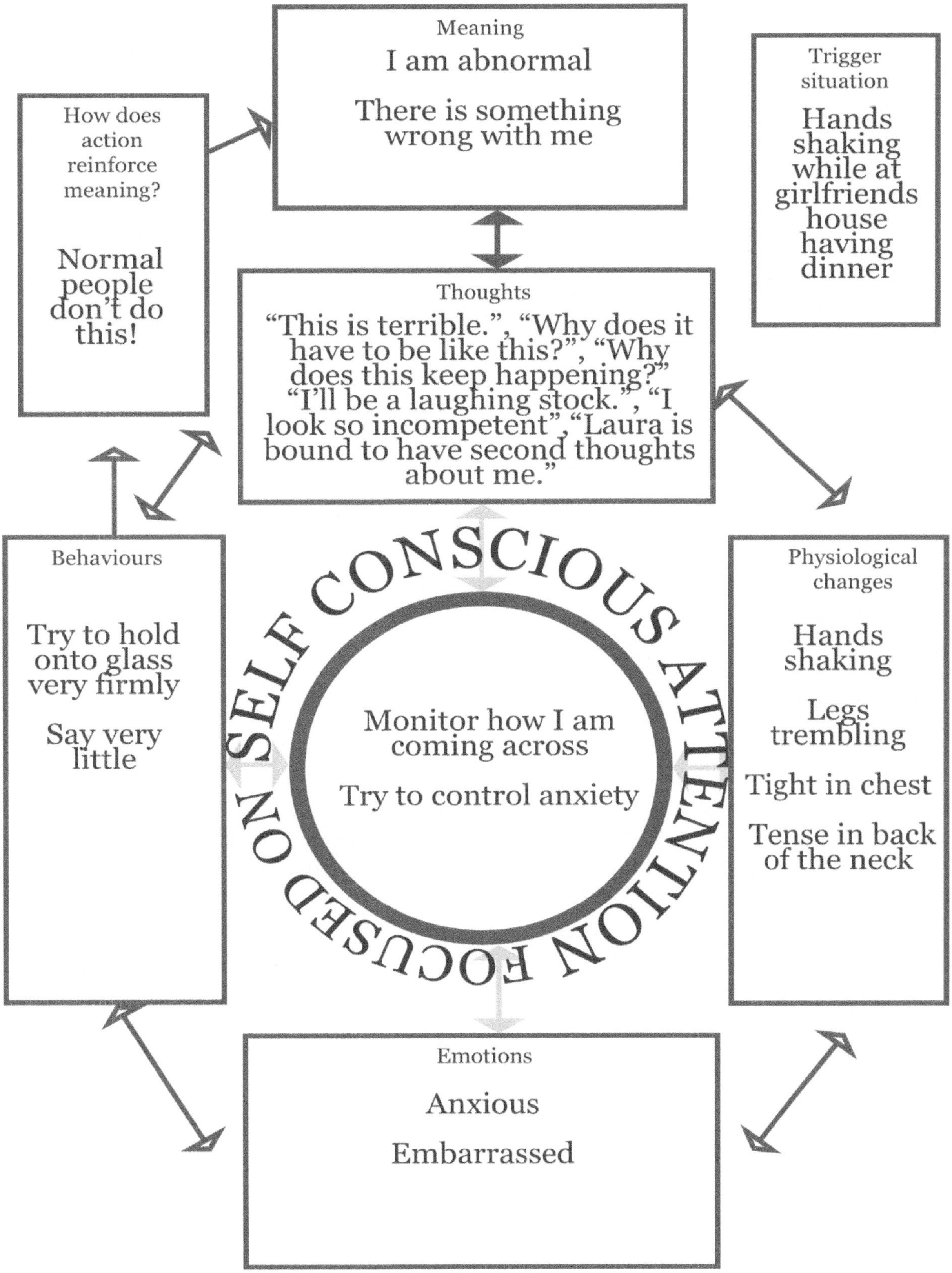

Figure 12. Social anxiety cycle

known as structural magnetic resonance imagery (MRI) - a type of brain scan - to measure the hippocampal sizes of participating taxi drivers. She found that London taxi drivers had significantly larger hippocampi than matched non-taxi drivers of a similar level of intelligence and driving experience, and the more experience a taxi driver had, the larger their hippocampus was. Eleanor Maguire's results were ground-breaking to the world of psychology as they demonstrated that there was the potential to grow and strengthen any brain area through the use of cognitive exercise.

Further advice on using thought diaries

If you find that using thought diaries acts as a trigger for you to mull things over too much then you are best off discontinuing using thought diaries, initially. You can return to them later on when you have learned how to use other cognitive exercises - covered later in this book. You may also find that you are not able to complete thought records when you feel really distressed. This is completely normal. If you feel that you can't complete a thought record when you are feeling really anxious, take out a thought record later (when you feel less distressed) and remind yourself about what happened.

Thought, feeling/physiology and behaviour diaries

When you compete self-observation diaries (see tables, 6, 7 & 8) they will a) provide useful material that you can work with and b) act as a low level CBT exercise.

Generally, most of us live our lives automatically, without giving much thought to a) thinking about our thinking, b) how we react to our feelings or c) what makes us behave the way that we do. Completing a thought diary brings more of these automatic processes into your awareness. Once these patterns are brought into your conscious awareness, you immediately have more choice about how to react. This is due to the fact that writing information down encourages a process of stepping back and observing. This type of detachment will automatically encourage the use of self-reflection. As soon as you start to consider what makes you think, feel, or behave the way that you do, you will be 'working out' the pre-frontal cortex, which can often disengage with anxiety.

Table 4. Thoughts, physiology, emotion and behaviour diary

Automatic thoughts, e.g. "She doesn't like me"	**Physiology, e.g. chest tightening**	**Emotion, e.g. anxiety**	**Behaviour, e.g. avoid contact with that person**

Table 4. Thoughts, physiology, emotion and behaviour diary

Automatic thoughts, e.g. "She doesn't like me"	**Physiology, e.g. chest tightening**	**Emotion, e.g. anxiety**	**Behaviour, e.g. avoid contact with that person**

Table 4. Thoughts, physiology, emotion and behaviour diary

Automatic thoughts, e.g. "She doesn't like me"	Physiology, e.g. chest tightening	Emotion, e.g. anxiety	Behaviour, e.g. avoid contact with that person

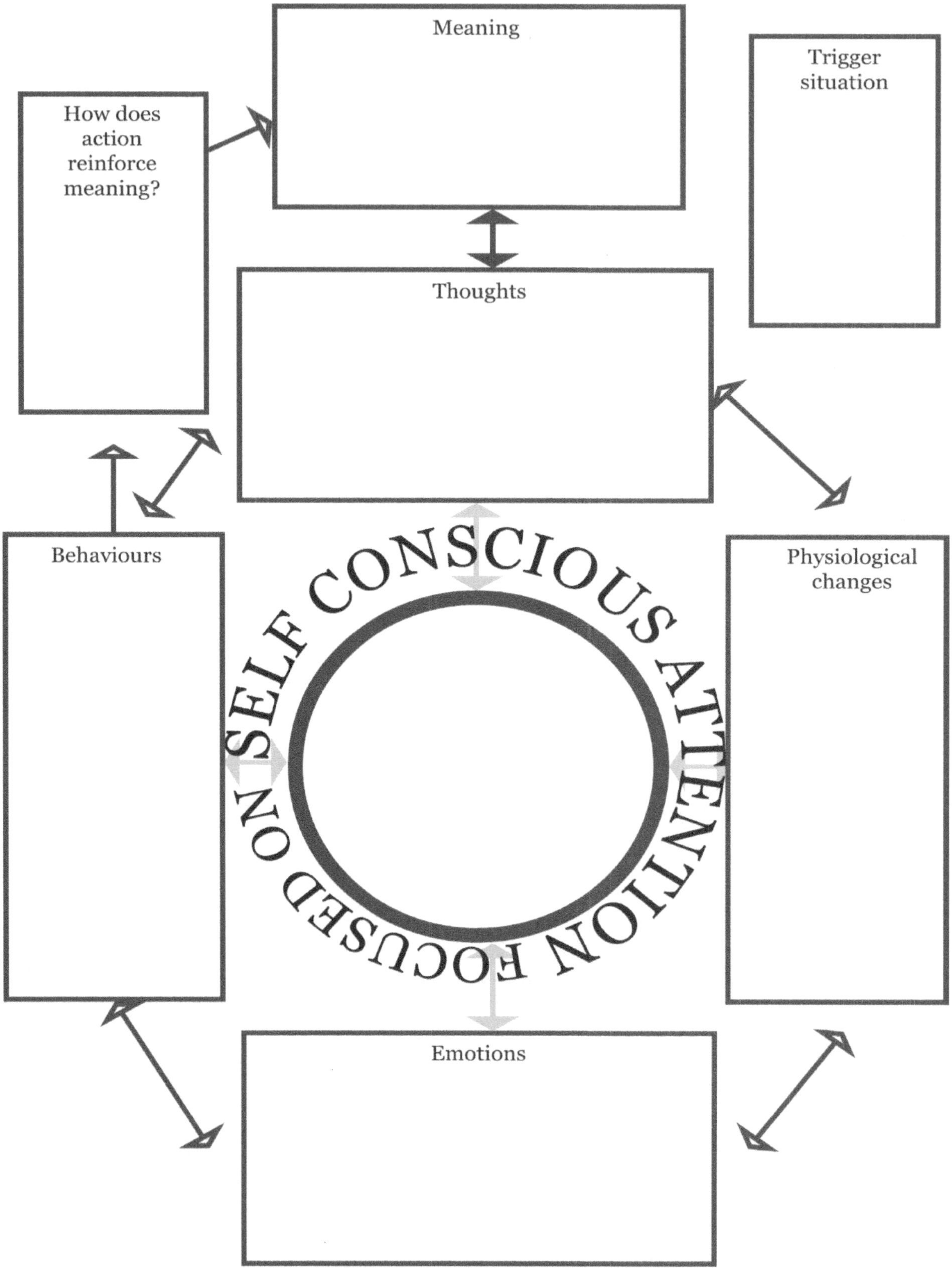

Figure 12. Social anxiety cycle

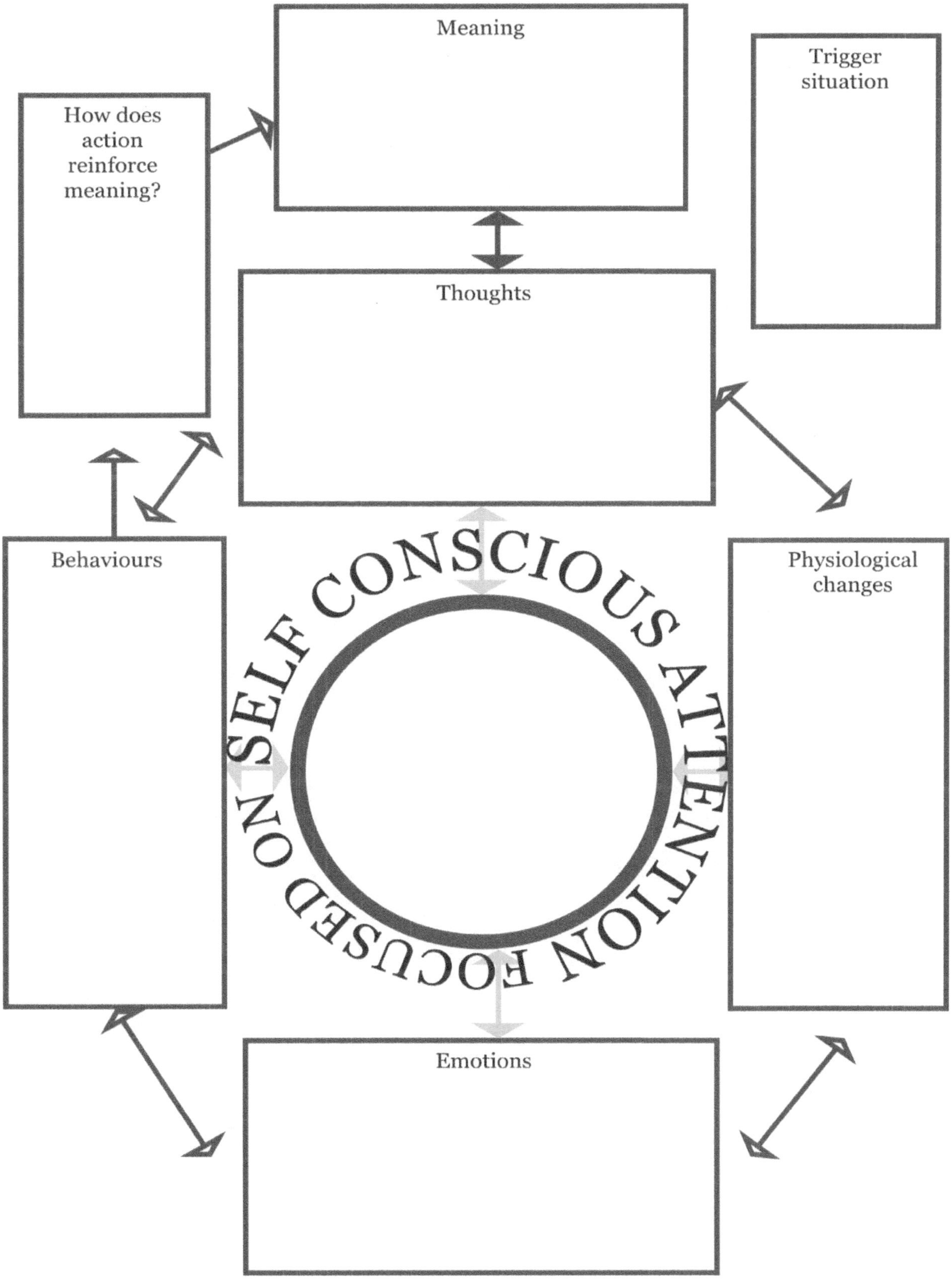

Figure 12. Social anxiety cycle

Table 5. Thought, physiology, emotion and behaviour sheet

Day: **Time:** **Trigger situation:**	**Thoughts:**

Physiological reactions

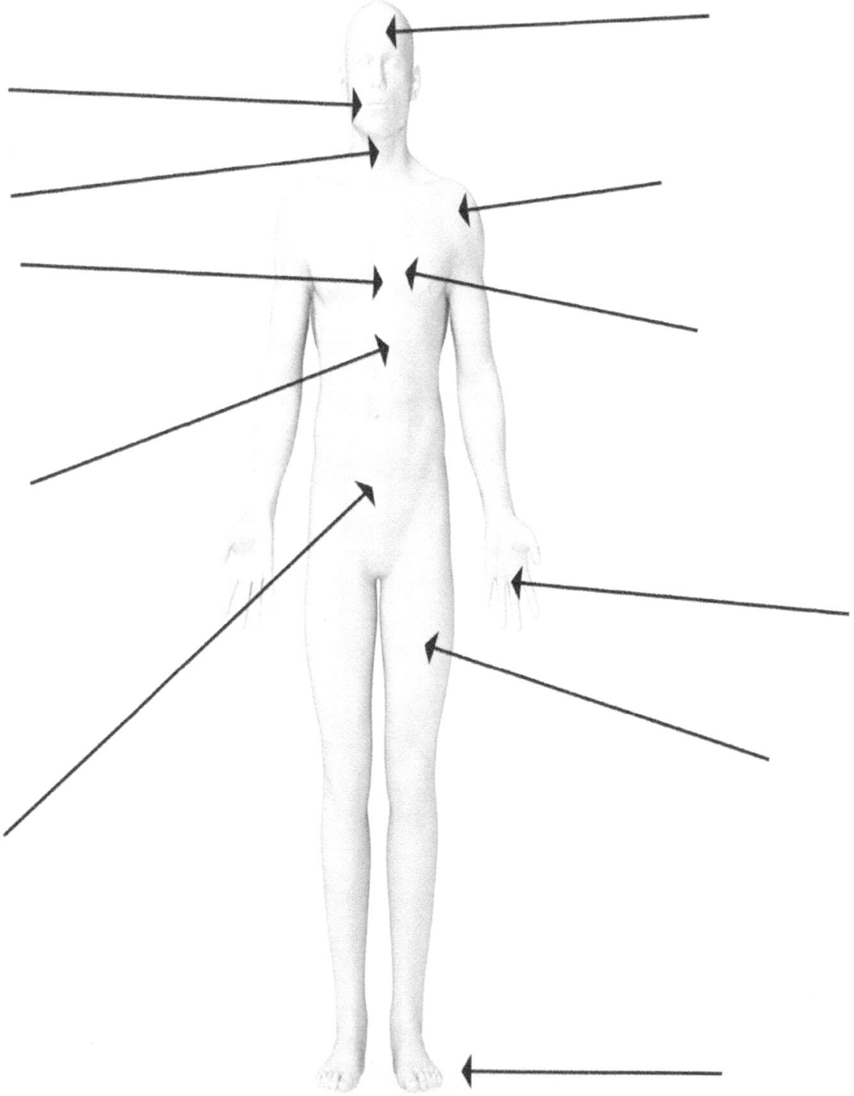

Emotion:	**Behaviour:**

Table 5. Thought, physiology, emotion and behaviour sheet

Day: **Time:** **Trigger situation:**	**Thoughts:**

Physiological reactions

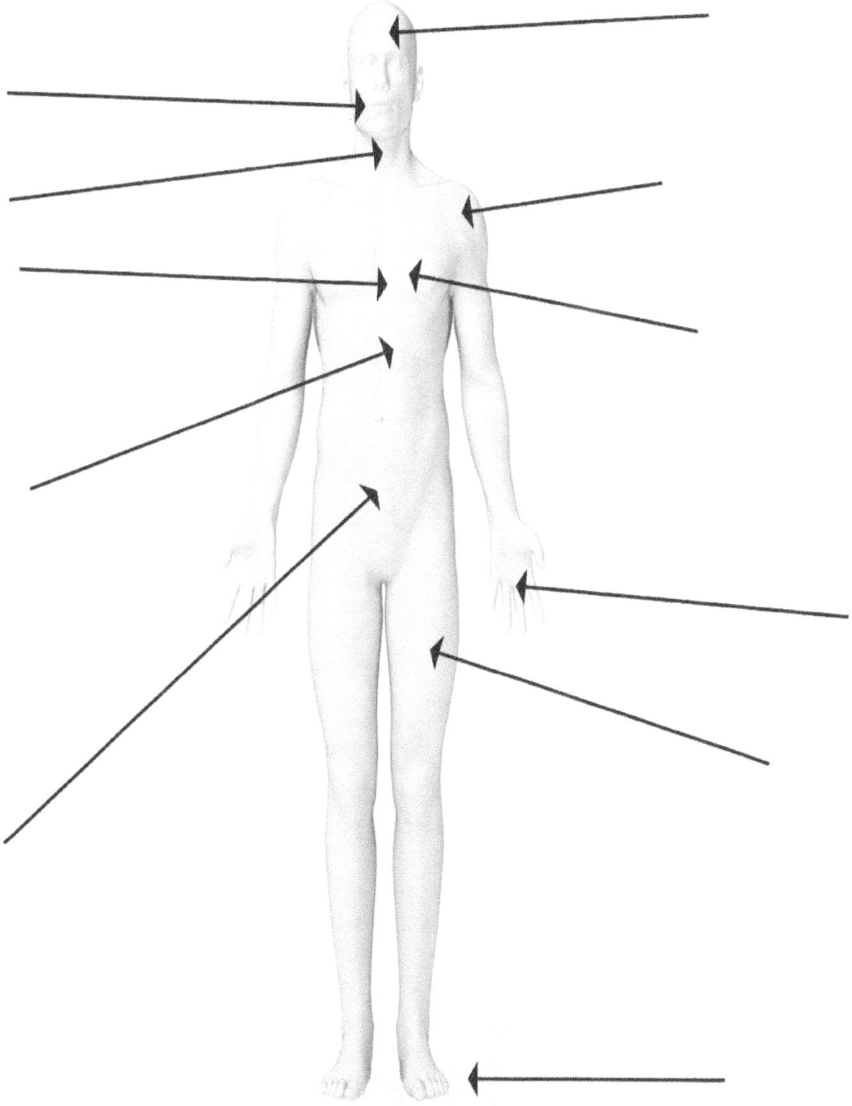

Emotion:	**Behaviour:**

Table 5. Thought, physiology, emotion and behaviour sheet

Day: **Time:** **Trigger situation:**	**Thoughts:**

Physiological reactions

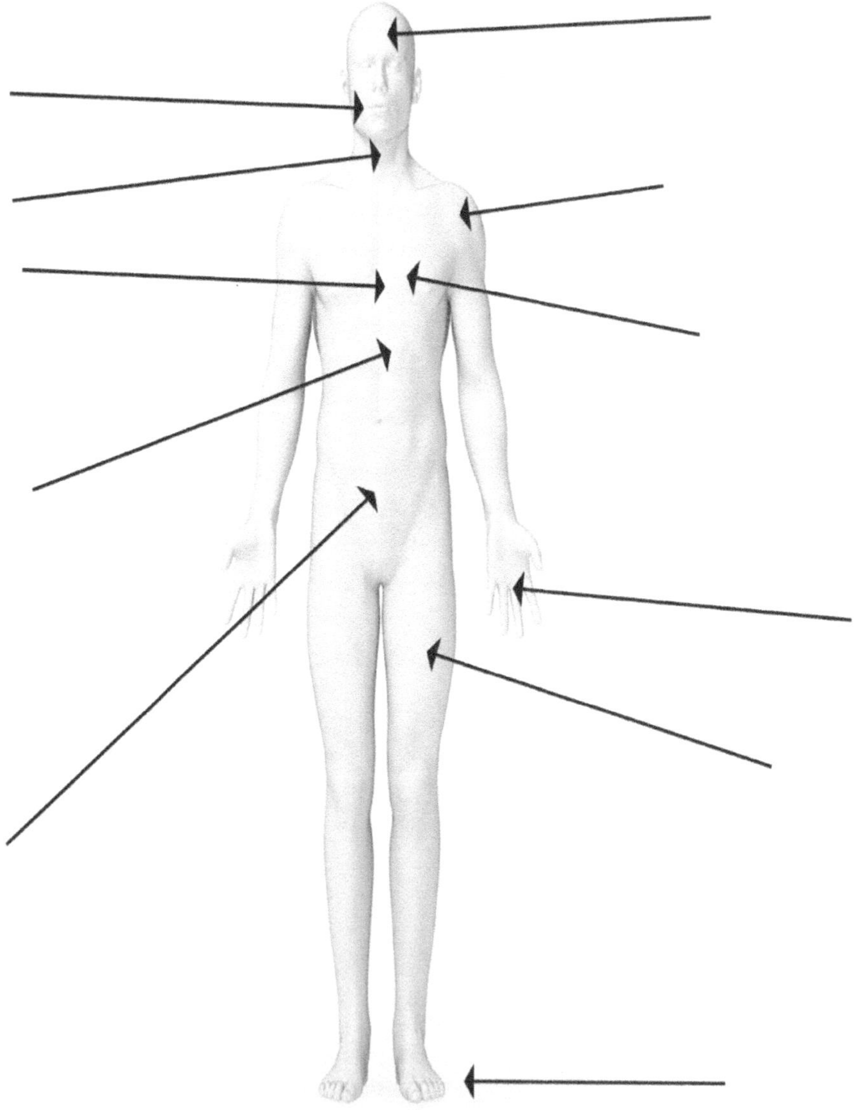

Emotion:	**Behaviour:**

Chapter summary
Observe yourself

- Self-observation increases your ability to stand back and think about your own thinking processes.

- Self-reflection is highly effortful for the mind, but importantly it can help to reduce your risk of relapsing in the future.

14 Rules

In my clinical work I often help my clients to identify the different types of rules that they hold. We all live by rules and most of the time our rules help us. They work automatically in the background of our minds helping us to make our way through cultural conventions and social occasions. We have literally hundreds of rules that guide our behaviour, for example, rules about queuing up, the way we drive our car, what to do when we attend a dinner party, how to use a knife and fork, what clothing to wear on what occasion, etc. Most of the time we are completely unaware of our rules unless someone breaks them; for example, if somebody pushes in front of us in a queue, talks out loud in a library, and so on.

Many of us also have rules that we use to protect ourselves from our deepest fears; for example, "If I come across as confident and in control, then I will be OK", "If I feel strong, and in control at all times, then I will be OK."

When I had my CBT I discovered my rules were mainly about how I wanted others to think of me. They were a bit of a surprise to me when I noticed them. I kind of knew they were there in the background but hadn't really thought about them in that way before. My rules were something along the lines of: "If I produce results and I am contributing at all times then I will be OK." And: "If I meet the highest standards at all times then I will be OK." My rules meant that I spent most of my time working and not spending time with my family. If I wasn't working, I felt as though something wasn't quite right. I found it difficult to stop and rest even for five minutes. If I stopped working I felt guilty or anxious. It felt wrong if I wasn't achieving something.

The development of rules

Rules are usually created early in our lives as children and they often help us during that period of time. However, as we grow older, rules can become out of date and **maladaptive**. By maladaptive I mean that our rules can hold us back rather than work for us. If you would like to investigate what your rules are, begin by noticing what you expect from yourself and others. I have placed some examples of rules that some people expect of themselves and others over the next two pages (see tables 6 & 7). If you are having one-to-one CBT it is usually a good idea to identify what your rules are with your therapist. Use the self (see table 6) and others (see table 7) rule lists to make a note of your rules. Rules about the self could be ideas such as "If others are happy with me at all times then I will be OK." Whereas, rules about others could be "If people respect me and listen to me then I will be OK."

Sometimes rules are difficult to recognise. Close friends and family members will help you to notice what your rules are if you ask them. I have put some of my rules below. If when you read them you think that my rules made me particularly difficult to live with and work with, you would be correct. I tended to get irritated, anxious, and angry if my rules were broken, often making life difficult for others as well as myself.

"If nobody is upset with me and everybody likes me at all times then I will be OK"

"If I work hard and achieve at all times then I will be OK"

"If I am in control at all times then I will be OK"

"If I am strong at all times then I will be OK"

"If people are happy with my performance then I will be OK"

"If I am the best at what I do then I will be OK"

"If people don't let me down then I will be OK"

During the time that I struggled the most I took on very difficult tasks and generally worked until I became exhausted. When I wasn't able to work the way I did before I felt guilty about not working and started beating myself up over it. In therapy, when I thought about what was happening it really brought my attention to what I was doing. I thought I was doing all the extra work to help others and my family but obviously it didn't feel that way to them. Ironically, in my valiant attempts to prove to myself that I was OK, I ended up upsetting most of the people that I came into contact with.

You can challenge your rules using CBT exercises (see table 8).

Table 6. Rules **(Use the box to the right to note which rules apply to you)**	✓
If I am in control at all times then I will be OK	
If people are happy with me at all times then I will be OK	
If I do things perfectly at all times then I will be OK	
If I am the best at what I do at all times then I will be OK	
If I don't experience any any unusual bodily sensations then I will be OK	
If I am feeling good at all times then I will be OK	
If I am feeling confident at all times then I will be OK	
If I am not blamed for things then I will be OK	
If I show dominance at all times then I will be OK	
If I perform well at all times then I will be OK	
If I am physically well at all times then I will be OK	
If I am assertive at all times then I will be OK	
If I know what I am doing at all times then I will be OK	
If I know what is going to happen at all times then I will be OK	
If I appear to others as though I know what I am doing then I will be OK	
If I feel safe at all times then I will be OK	
If I appear competent at all times then I will be OK	
If I show no signs of vulnerability then I will be OK	
If I am in control of my feelings at all times then I will be OK	
If I say "Yes" to all requests at all times then I will be OK	
If I am strong at all times then I will be OK	
If things go wrong it is all my fault	
If I don't let people down then I will be OK	
If I can fix things then I will be OK	
If I am in control of my body at all times then I will be OK	
Total number of rules endorsed (write number of rules endorsed in right-hand column).	

Table 7. Rules for others **(Use the box to the right to note which rules apply to you)**	✓
If others don't challenge me then I will be OK	
If people are happy with me at all times then I will be OK	
If people around me don't make any mistakes then I will be OK	
If others tell me that I am the best at what I do at all times then I will be OK	
If people around me are happy, calm and relaxed, then I will be OK	
If people around me are polite and respectful then I will be OK	
If people around me are confident then I will be OK	
If others don't criticise me then I will be OK	
If others let me take charge then I will be OK	
If people around me approeciate me then I will be OK	
If people around tell me that I am alright then I will be OK	
If people listen to me at all times then I will be OK	
If people around me know what they are doing at all times then I will be OK	
If others reassure me then I will be OK	
If others show confidence in me at all times then I will be OK	
If others help me feel safe then I will be OK	
If others approve of me at all times then I will be OK	
If others show no signs of vulnerability then I will be OK	
If others put my needs ahead of their own then I will be OK	
If others say "Yes" to my requests when I ask them, then I will be OK	
If I am around strong people then I will be OK	
If others take the blame for mistakes then I wil be OK	
If others don't let me down then I will be OK	
If others can fix things for me then I will be OK	
If others are there for me when I need them then I will be OK	
Total number of rules endorsed (write number of rules endorsed in right-hand column).	

Table 8. Rule challenging exercise

Rule

How real and familiar does this rule feel?

What impact does the rule have on your life?

What benefits does this rule have on your life?

Were you born with that rule?

How old is the rule?

Where do you think this rule came from?

If you learnt the rule from a person where do you think he or she learnt it from?

Do you want to keep this rule?

If you gave yourself an opportunity to have another rule, what rule would you pick?

How do you think you might feel if you choose to live by your new rule as much as you did the old one?

How does knowing that you can choose to have another rule make you feel?

Table 8. Rule challenging exercise

Rule	How old is the rule?	If you gave yourself an opportunity to have another rule, what rule would you pick?
How real and familiar does this rule feel?	Where do you think this rule came from?	How do you think you might feel if you choose to live by your new rule as much as you did the old one?
What impact does the rule have on your life?	If you learnt the rule from a person where do you think he or she learnt it from?	How does knowing that you can choose to have another rule make you feel?
What benefits does this rule have on your life?	Do you want to keep this rule?	
Were you born with that rule?		

Table 8. Rule challenging exercise

Rule	How old is the rule?	If you gave yourself an opportunity to have another rule, what rule would you pick?
How real and familiar does this rule feel?	Where do you think this rule came from?	How do you think you might feel if you choose to live by your new rule as much as you did the old one?
What impact does the rule have on your life?	If you learnt the rule from a person where do you think he or she learnt it from?	How does knowing that you can choose to have another rule make you feel?
What benefits does this rule have on your life?	Do you want to keep this rule?	
Were you born with that rule?		

Chapter summary
Rules

- We initially develop rules to keep ourselves safe.
- Rules can be difficult to recognise and many of us are unaware that we have them.
- When our rules are broken we usually experience an emotional reaction.

15 Beliefs

Generally speaking, limiting beliefs are deeply held ideas about ourselves that we fear are true. By the time that we become adults, our beliefs can become so set within us that we feel that they are part of who we are. We may also carry out numerous 'safety behaviours' to protect ourselves from them without being aware of it. Most of us have absolutely no idea that our beliefs are running us.

I discovered that one of my limiting beliefs was: "I am a failure!" The funny thing about it was no matter how hard I worked or how much I achieved, the belief "I am a failure" was always still there. It seemed like what I had done in the past counted for nothing. Trying to prove the belief wrong demanded so much of my time that it affected my health and the happiness of my family. I didn't realise it was driving me so much. I didn't feel in control of my life. It drove me to do more and more. I didn't really know how to stop! My CBT therapist helped me to notice that in many situations I was experiencing high levels of painful emotions that were inconsistent with the situation that I was faced with. For example, we identified that I had an over-the-top reaction to even small amounts of criticism. Using this awareness my therapist helped me to recognise that the belief "I am a failure" which was experienced at a 'felt sense level' was the main driver for my emotional reaction. My extreme distress response was the primitive part of my brain trying to protect me from being a failure.

After this, I became much more observant and aware of my emotional reactions (without judging them) and I usually took a minute out to see if a limiting belief was influencing me. When I became distressed my thinking may have gone something along the lines of: "That's interesting! I'm experiencing really intense feelings right now, but I haven't actually done anything wrong and nothing is going to happen to me. What am I possibly stuck with right now or believing about myself that is making me feel this way?"

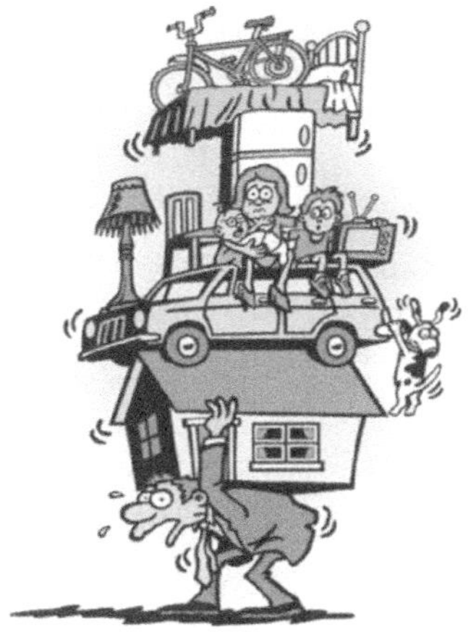

"James! Do you think you might be trying to do too much again?"

How do we develop limiting beliefs?

The most obvious ways that we develop limiting beliefs do not really need any scientific evidence or scientific explanation. If parents or caregivers tell their children that they are weak, stupid, worthless, or a failure it is purely logical that most children will develop limiting beliefs! Most of us would understand that children treated in this way would develop a negative view of themselves. In a similar manner, children can develop limiting beliefs through negative messages from care givers that are implied through action and inaction. Once a child develops limiting beliefs they are usually very difficult to shift and tend to be retained into adulthood.

There are also other ways in which people develop beliefs: ways we might not normally think about. I am saying this because I have come across a large number of clients who appear to have limiting beliefs, yet they cannot recall any significant trauma, and they have no history of parental abuse or poor treatment in their childhood.

The subtle ways that we develop beliefs

In 2014, researchers from the University of Michigan, Jacek Debiec and Regina Sullivan completed some interesting research on rats. They taught young female rats to fear the smell of peppermint by pumping the smell of peppermint into their cages and giving them electric shocks at the same time. The female rats were then left to their own devices for a while, mated, became pregnant, and gave birth. After the mothers had given birth researchers re-exposed the mother rats to the peppermint smell again, without electric shocks this time, while they were with their young. The researchers found that infant rats learned to fear the peppermint smell by noticing the scent of fear given off by their mothers. Brain scans carried out on the baby rats revealed that a fear of peppermint was programmed directly into the infant rats' amygdala. As I wrote about earlier, the amygdala is the seat of our natural response to threat. There is growing evidence that infant children's brains operate in a similar way to baby rats' brains, both in the womb and after birth up until the age of 6 months. Research in this area is still being carried out.

Research findings such as those described above are beginning to suggest at a most basic level that children absorb their parents' fears. The implication is that we are biologically pre-programed to accept a rapid transfer or download of information from our parents. One of the reasons why Jacek Debiec set up his experiments in the first place was because he had come across many people who came to him with nightmares and post-traumatic symptoms connected to the Holocaust. The issue that confused him most of all was that these particular adults with post-trauma symptoms had not even been born during the Holocaust; they were children of Holocaust survivors and somehow and someway they had absorbed the fears of their parents.

Social learning and belief systems

The above methods of learning belief systems are not the only ways that we can develop belief systems. There is also a process called social learning that we will need to give some attention to.

In 1977, Albert Bandura wrote about a process he identified in children called observational learning, which is now more commonly known as social learning theory: He witnessed that children act as little information processers watching and copying the behaviour of important others, or role models. In this respect, you are highly likely to develop the fears/beliefs of care-givers.

Identifying limiting beliefs in CBT

To identify limiting beliefs I usually begin by asking my clients to remember a situation where they experienced quite intense emotions. Clients determine if their emotion is more intense than they think is appropriate for their situation. I then help my clients to complete a CBT exercise called a **downward arrow**. With a downward arrow exercise, therapists help their clients to keep following feelings and thoughts until their clients reach the deepest fears that they hold about themselves. I have put an example of a downward arrow exercise on the next page (see table 9).

I strongly advise you not to do this exercise by yourself unless you have already completed CBT with a trained therapist.

Table 9. **Downward arrow exercise**

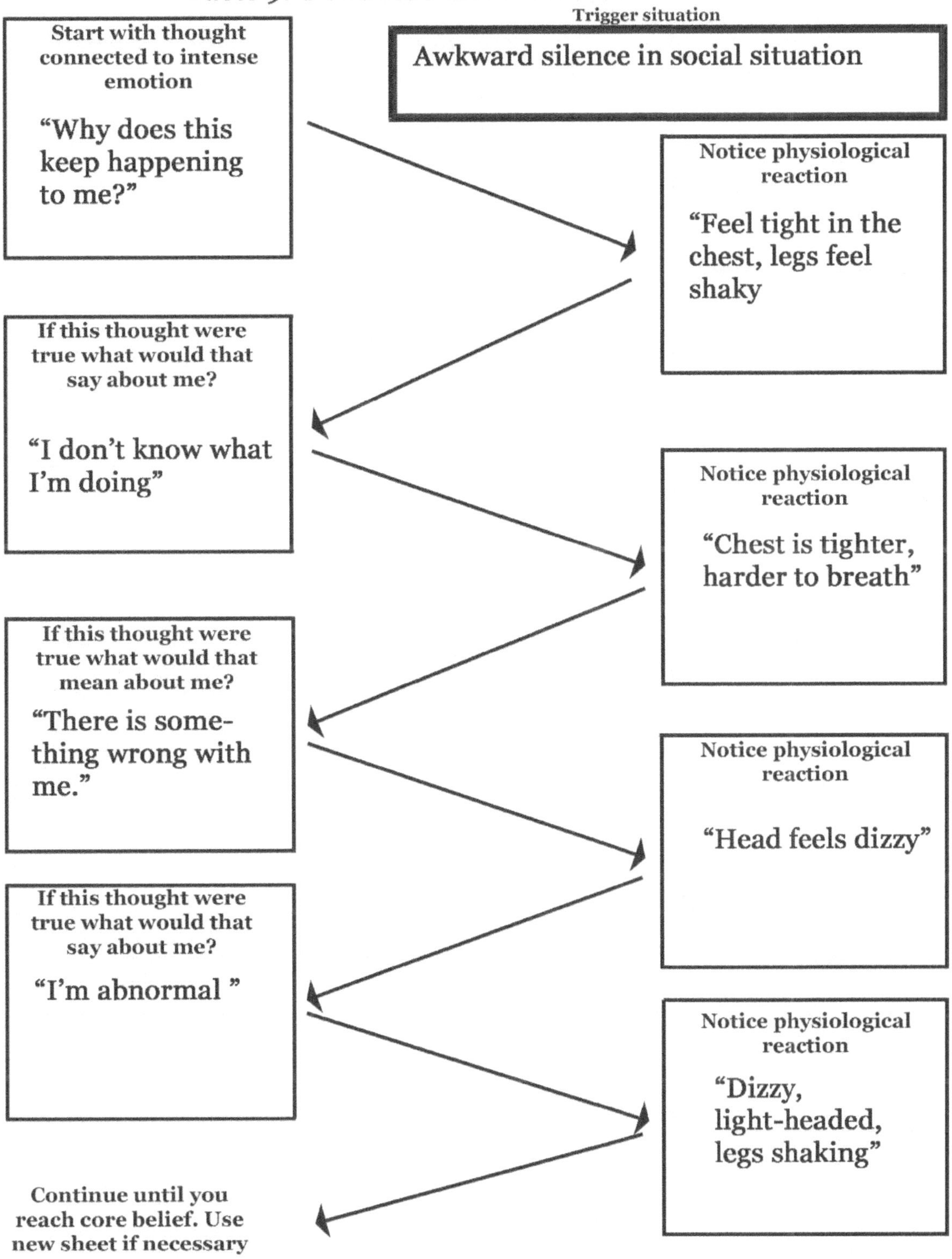

Downward arrow exercise

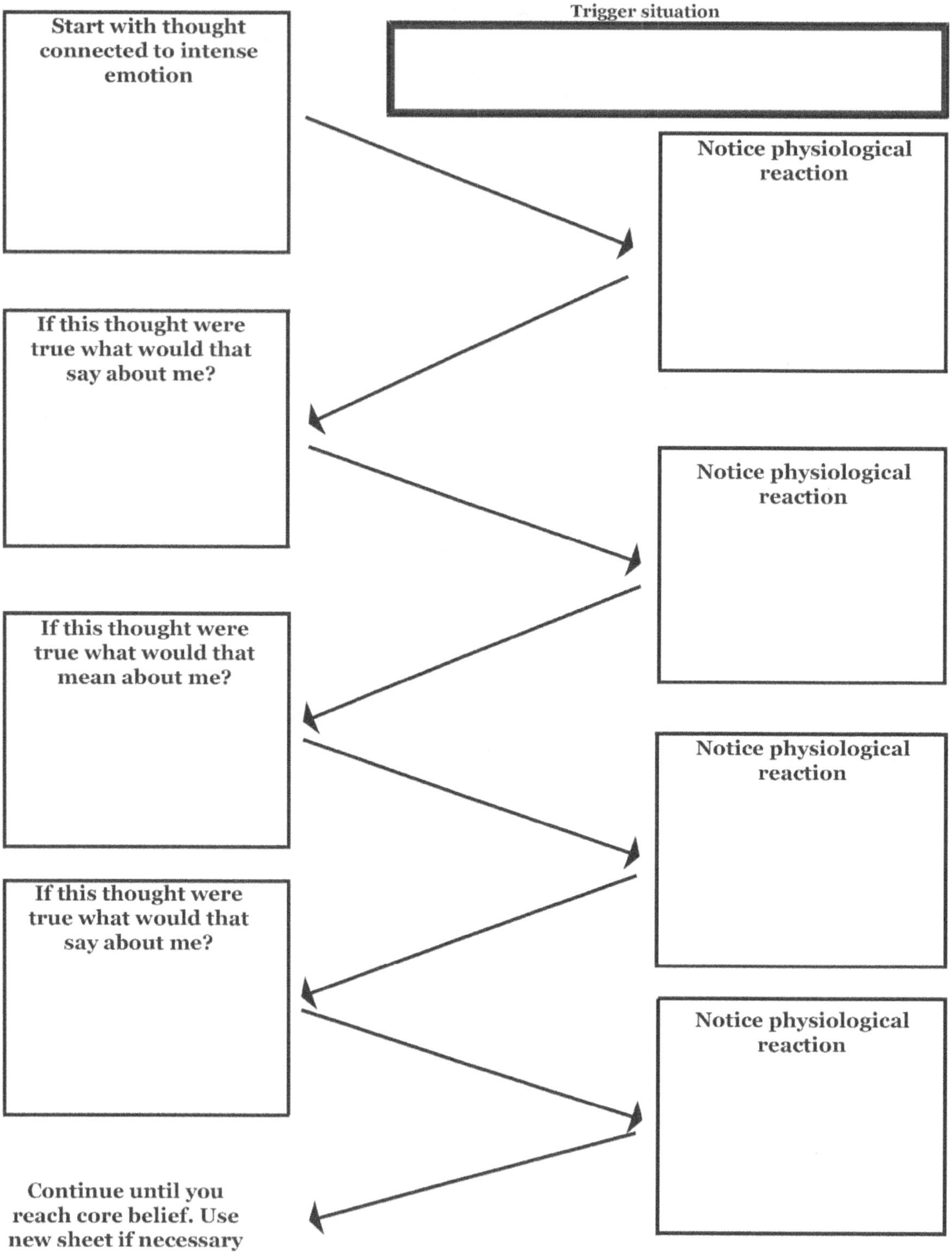

Downward arrow exercise

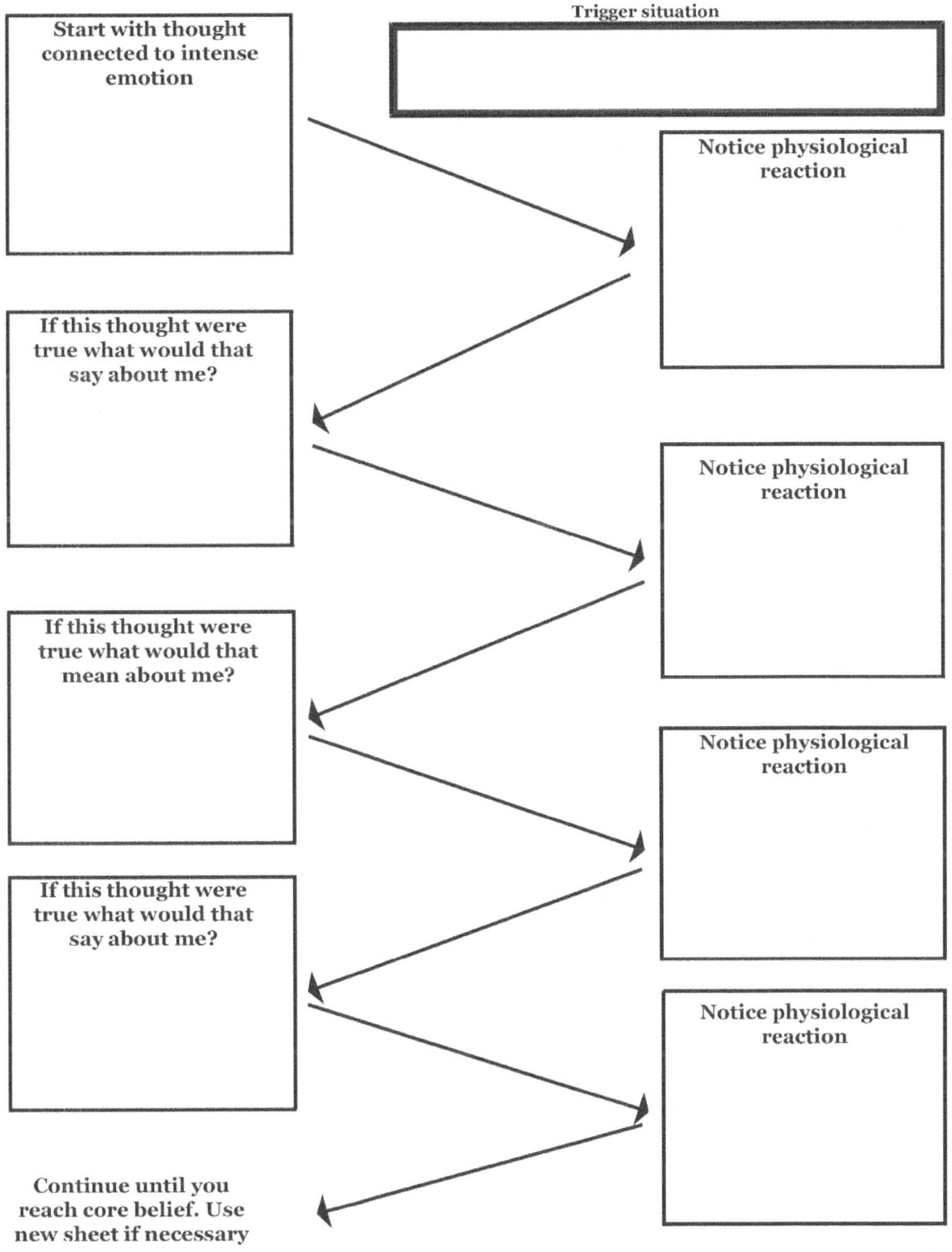

Downward arrow exercise

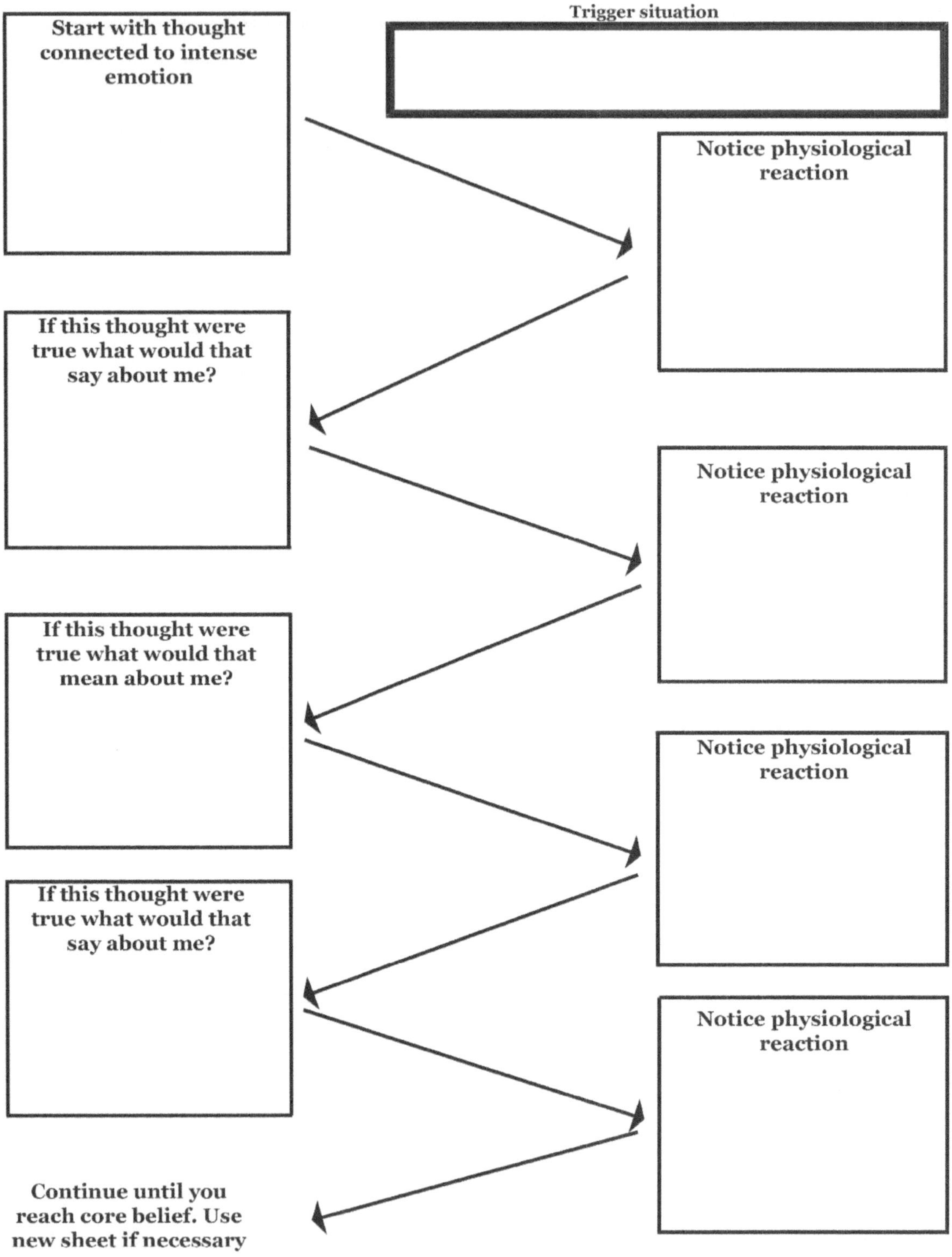

Chapter summary

Beliefs

- Beliefs are deeply held ideas about the self that we fear are true.
- Beliefs tend to be developed in childhood and we carry them into adult life.
- A downward arrow exercise is often used to identify beliefs in CBT.

16 Drawing out CBT cycles

In my sessions with clients I often draw out cycles using my whiteboard to explain how people's distressing feelings and behaviours are being maintained. A general idea behind drawing out cycles is to help people recognise that some of the things that they do tend to keep their problems in place. Once you realise that you have a cycle in place, you will then need to work out how to break the cycle.

There are several ways to draw out cycles. I'd like us to start with making a connection between beliefs, rules, and safety behaviours. A CBT cycle for social anxiety generally looks a bit like figure 13 on the next page.

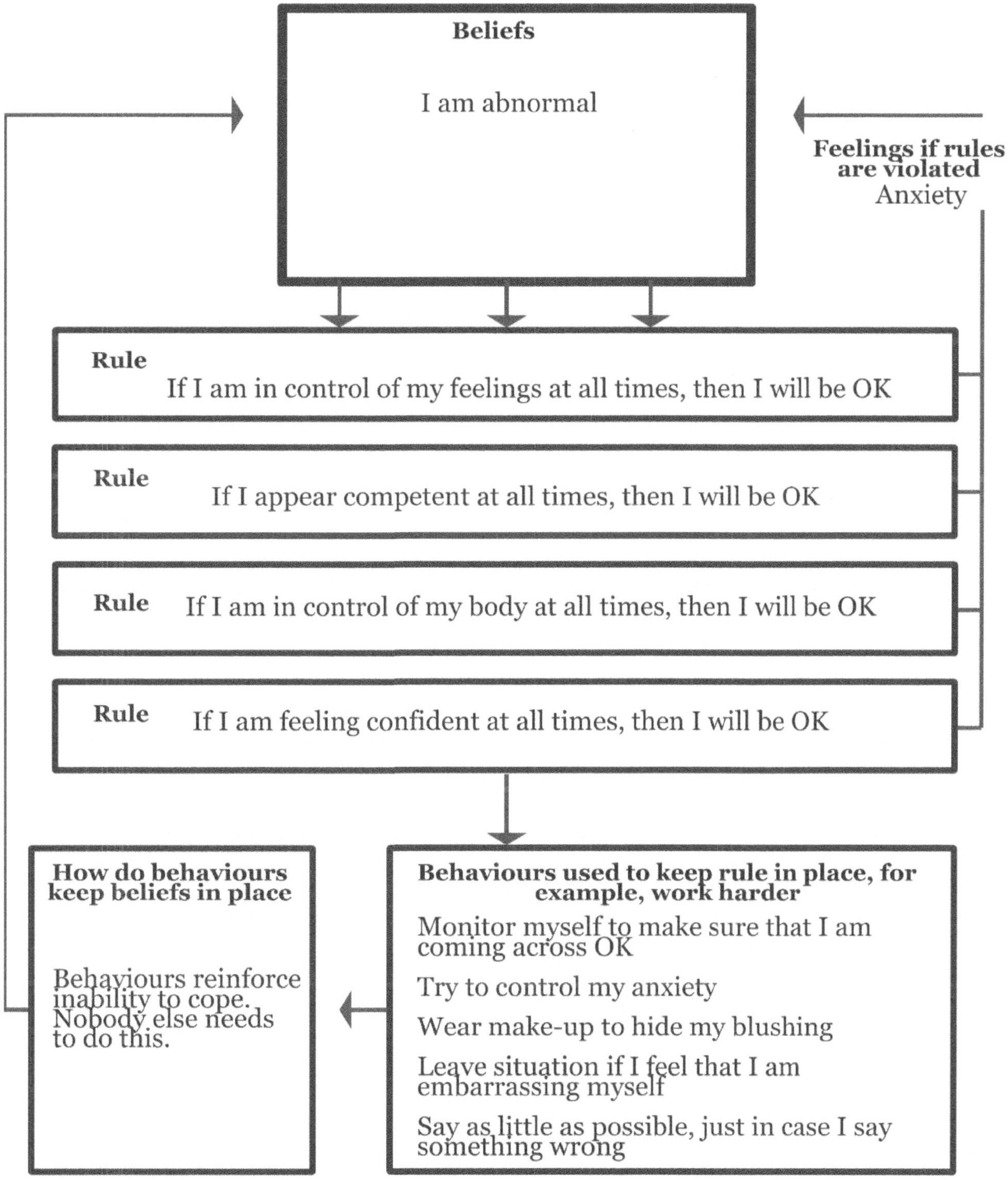

Figure 13. Cycle of beliefs, rules, and behaviours

Cycle of beliefs, rules, and behaviours

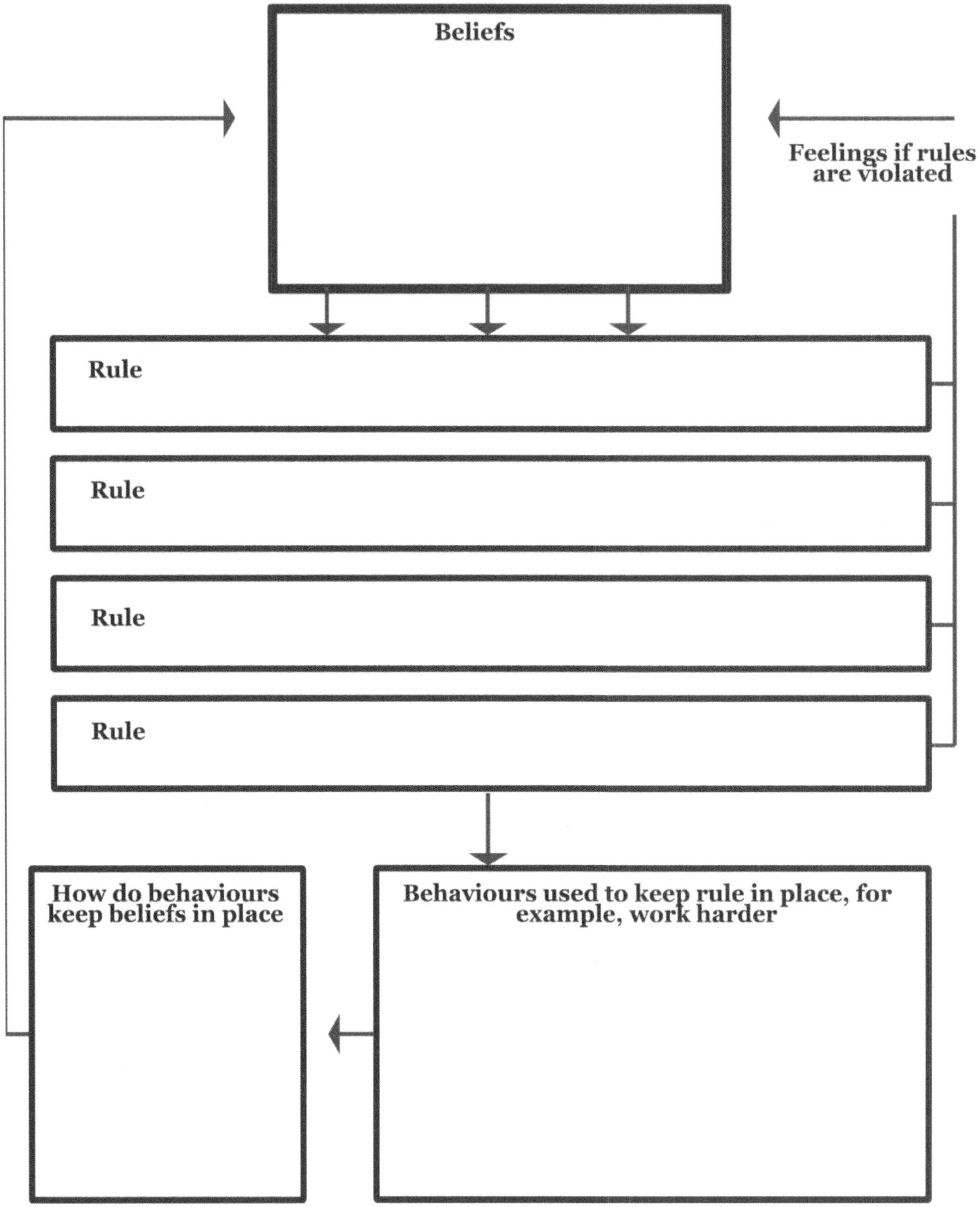

Chapter summary
Drawing out CBT cycles

- A CBT cycle can be created to connect beliefs, rules, and behaviours.
- CBT cycles can be very useful for demonstrating how self-fulfilling prophecies work.

17 Challenging NATs

A practice that many cognitive behaviour therapists teach is challenging NATs. As I mentioned earlier NATs are the types of thoughts that run in our minds when we feel panicky or anxious. NATs are important to identify in CBT because they affect the way that we feel. Because of this, it will be very important for you to notice and challenge them as early as possible.

The first stage in recognising NATs is to set aside some time before or after social events that provoke more intense anxiety and write down the types of frightening automatic thoughts that come to mind. I have placed a list of common thoughts that people with social anxiety have below.

Common automatic thoughts in social anxiety

"People will find me boring"

"My shaking will give me away"

"People aren't interested in finding out what I have to say"

"People won't mind if I leave early"

"I look odd"

"I have nothing to contribute"

"People don't invite me anywhere"

"I look stupid"

"I have no social skills"

"They won't mind if I cancel, in fact they will be relieved"

"I am boring ...everyone is looking at me"

"I am making a fool of myself"

One of the most effective ways to challenge NATs is to bring them to awareness. Bringing NATs to awareness prevents them running automatically in the back of your minds, continually affecting the way that you feel.

What do you do with NATs after you bring them into awareness?

Stage 1. Once you recognise that you have NATs you then have a choice about how you decide to react to them. You can challenge them, or become aware of them and choose not to react to them. Many of my clients find that noticing their NATs and choosing not to react to them is very difficult, initially. With this in mind, I often find it useful in the early stages to spend time with my clients teaching them how to challenge their NATs. Ben, one of my clients had a NAT "I'll be a laughing stock". This was due to his hands shaking while he was at his girlfriends' parent's house. His Padesky cycle is on page 101, (see figure 14).

Stage 2. The second stage in challenging NATs is to bring alternative explanations to mind using a thought challenging record (see table 10). A thought challenging record is really a collection of notes that you can make to provide alternative evidence against your NATs. NATs are placed in the first column, evidence for the automatic thoughts are placed in the second column, evidence against the NAT is placed in the third column, and an alternative more balanced thought is placed in the fourth column.

Collecting evidence against NATs can sometimes be difficult and because of this it will be important to persist. Some people find it helpful to complete NAT challenging exercises with their therapist. Alternatively, you might ask trusted loved ones to help you challenge your NATs. You could also think about what you might say to others with similar problems to yourself if you were challenging their NATs.

Stage 3. After completing a thought challenging record it is often useful to put the alternative more balanced thought into a positive CBT cycle to look at how it might change things. Please see figure 15 for Ben's positive CBT cycle.

NB. NATs have a habit of coming back, so it may be useful for you to get your NAT challenging notes out and re-read them when this occurs.

Look out for cognitive distortions when you challenge your NATs

When we become distressed, the way that we think can change. High levels of distress can distort our perception, mood, and behaviour, directly affecting the way we make sense of things. When this occurs our thinking style can move from being balanced, flexible, expansive, and considering to a more rigid style (see chapter 11).

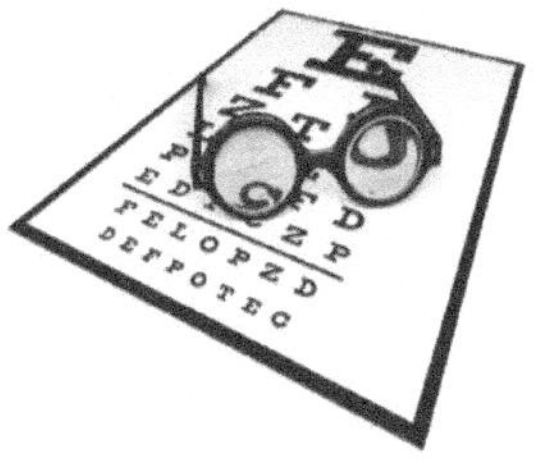

After having CBT sessions for a little while, I recognised the amount of cognitive distortions I had in my thinking. The best way I can think of to explain it is to imagine that someone puts some glasses on you, but you don't realise that you're wearing them. The glasses can make things seem much bigger or smaller than they really are.

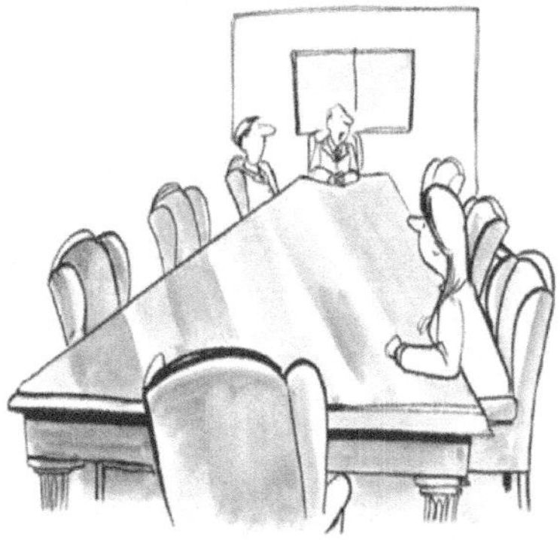

"I'm so glad that you could all make it today..."

When I began work with my therapist she helped me to realise that when I got upset I didn't always see the world clearly. Sometimes I filtered information so that I only saw what my mind would let me see. This meant I had a limited viewpoint and could not see what was really happening in my life!

At other times, I felt really sure that I knew what was going to happen before things actually happened.

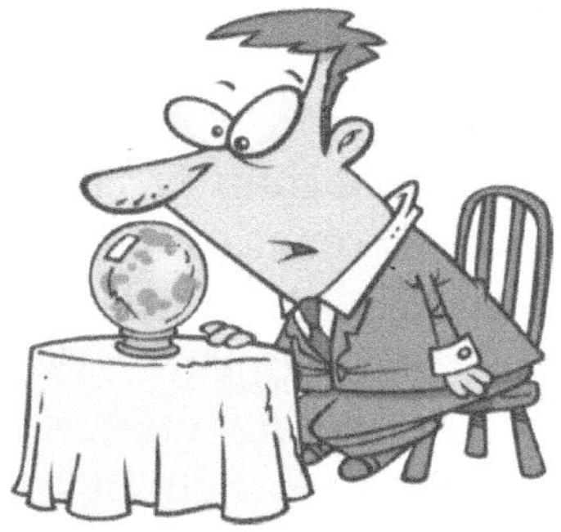

"Looks like it's going to be terrible tonight! I think I had better stay in."

And, everywhere I looked I could see danger.

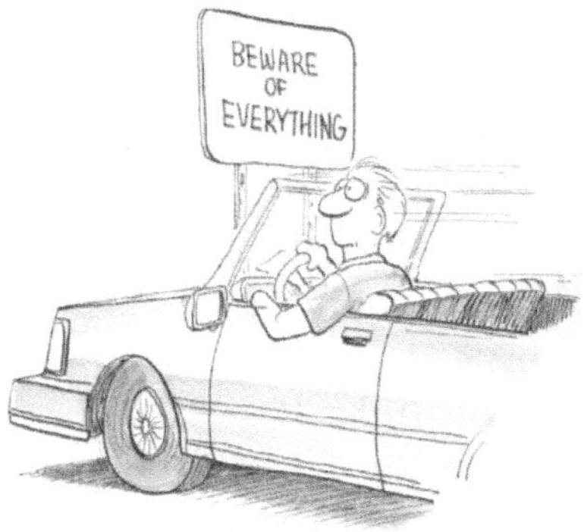

It is vital in your CBT journey that you learn to recognise when cognitive distortions are occurring so that as time progresses you can learn how to detach from them.

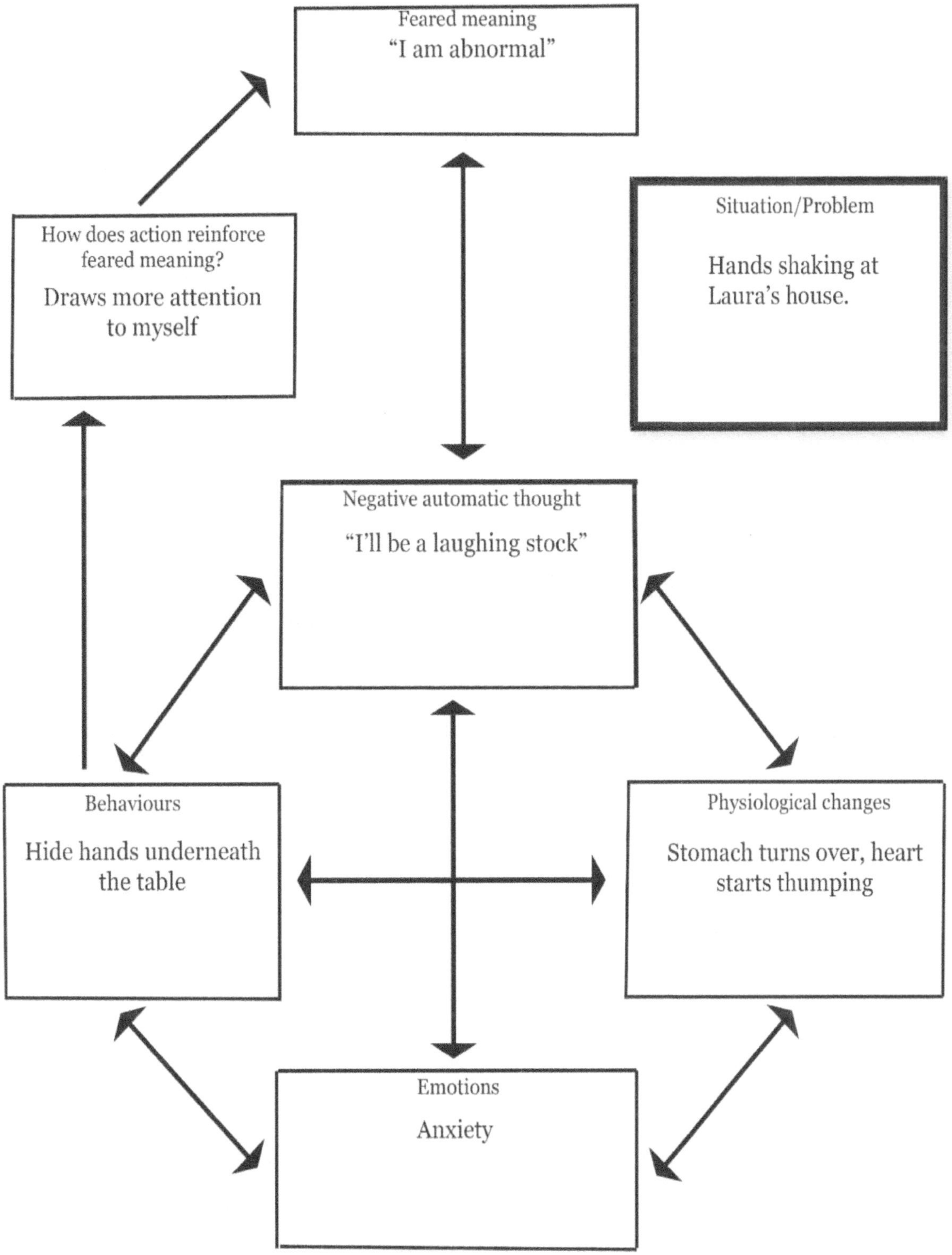

Figure 14. Maintenance cycle based on Christine Padesky's 'Hot-Cross Bun' approach

Table 10. NAT challenging form

Situation: Dinner with my girlfriend's parents. Hands shaking			
Negative automatic thoughts	Evidence for negative automatic thought	Alternative explanations	More balanced thought
"I'll be a laughing stock."	My brother pointed out that my hands were shaking a couple of years back and asked me what was happening. I have thoughts about people laughing and talking about me. It's not normal for people's hands to shake.	No one was laughing. Laura still wants to go out with me. I have never seen anybody laughing ever. Most people don't care or don't notice my hands shaking If somebody did point out that my hands were shaking it would probably say quite a lot about them, more than me.	More balanced thought "Yes I do get anxious, but most people don't seem to notice or they don't care."
"Laura is bound to have second thoughts about me."	It took quite a while for Laura to agree to go out with me. Laura might think I'm insecure and anxious and find that unattractive.	"Laura didn't mention anything. Laura's family were very friendly towards me. If Laura were to make those kind of judgements she isn't the girl I thought she was." "People don't think the same way that I do." "I may have other qualities that Laura likes about me."	More balanced thought "I do have doubts, as most teenagers do, but I've thought this several times before and nothing has happened."

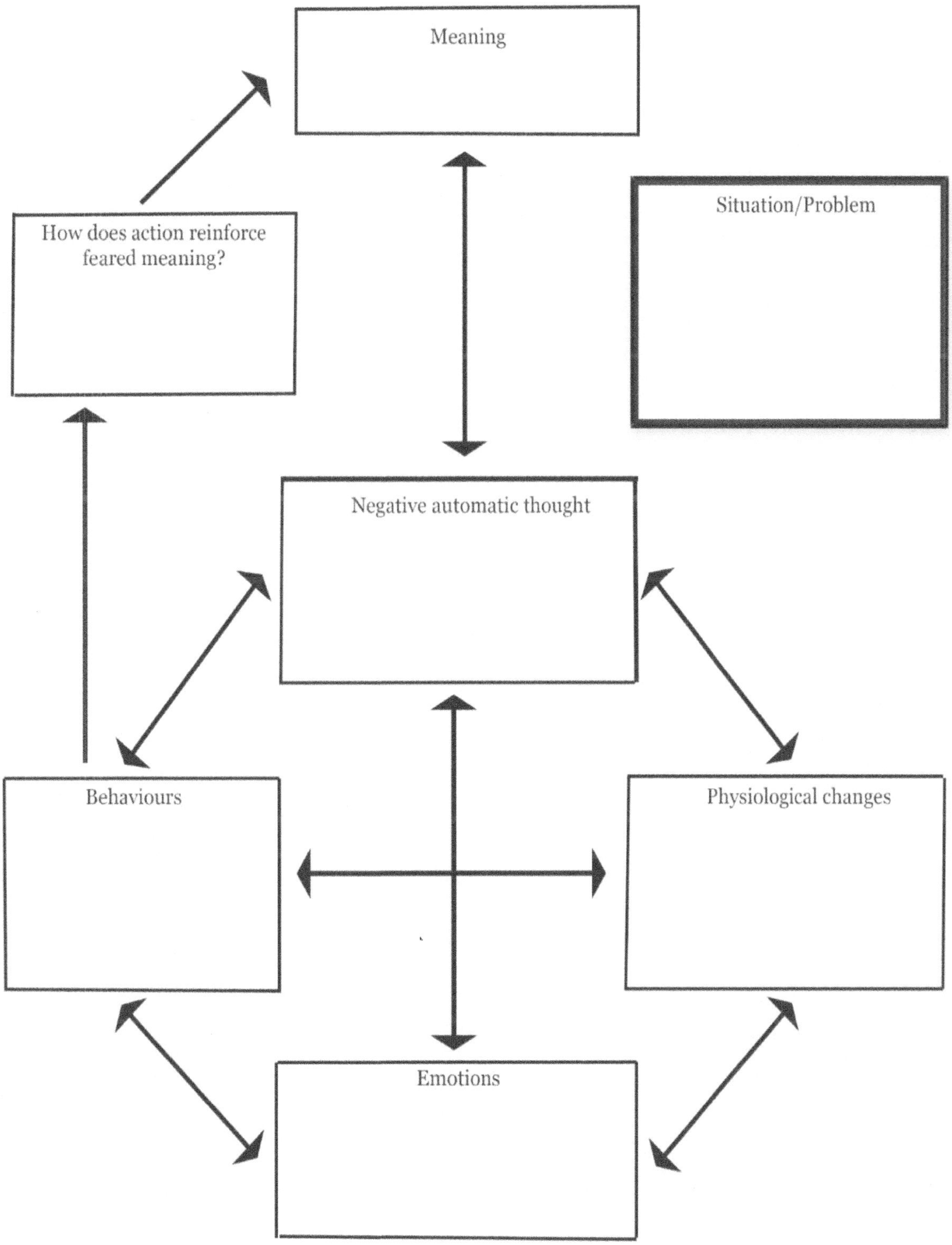

Figure 14. Negative maintenance cycle based on Christine Padesky's 'Hot-Cross Bun' approach

Table 11. NAT challenging form

Negative automatic thought, for example, "I will be a laughing stock!"	Evidence for negative automatic thought, for example, "I feel that it might happen"	Evidence against negative automatic thought, for example, this has never happened before	New more balanced thought, for example, although I feel anxious nothing has happened in the past and is unlikely to happen this time	How does creating a new more balanced thought affect the way that I feel, e.g., anxiety reduces

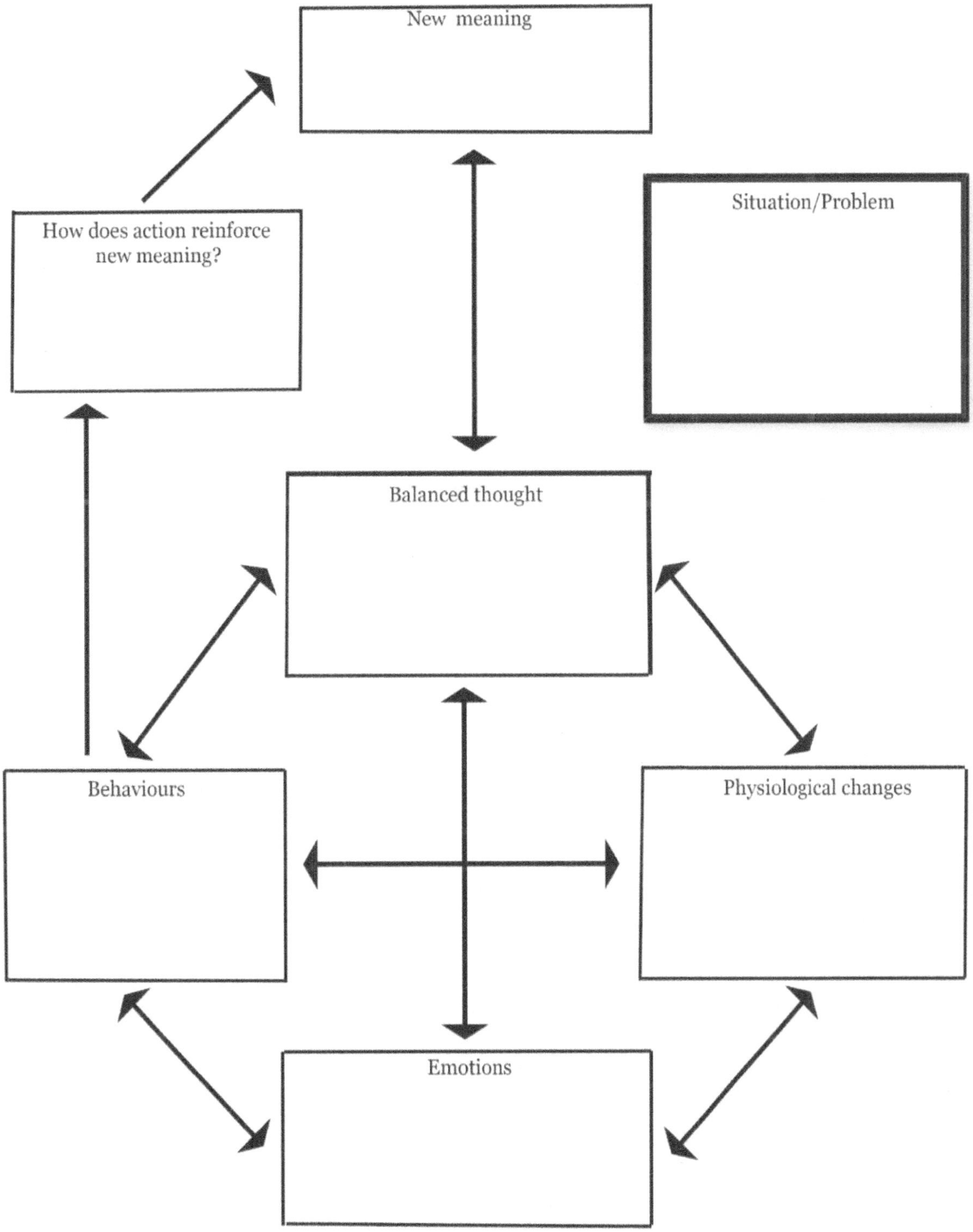

Figure 15. Positive maintenance cycle based on Christine Padesky's 'Hot-Cross Bun' approach

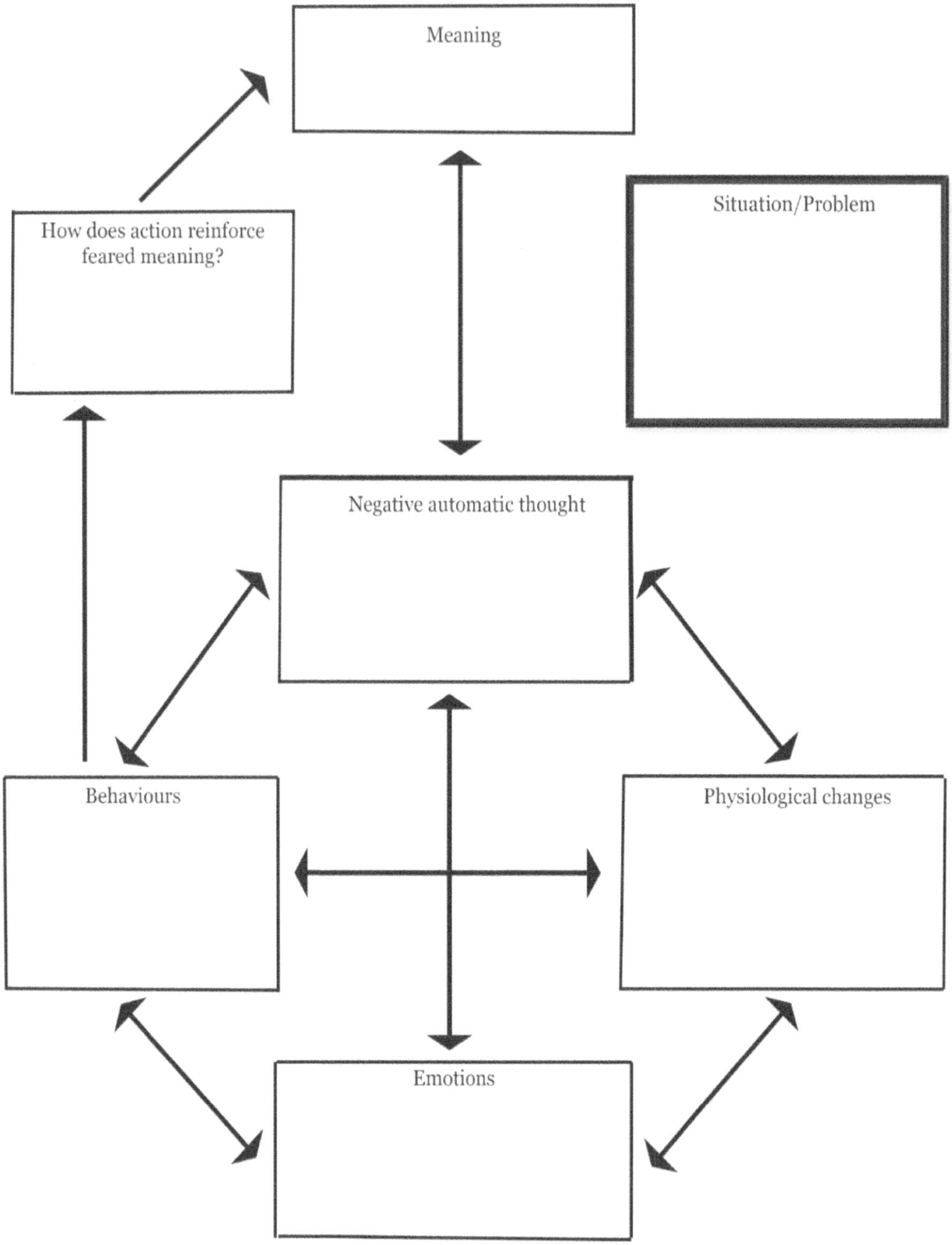

Figure 14. Negative maintenance cycle based on Christine Padesky's 'Hot-Cross Bun' approach

Table 11. NAT challenging form

Negative automatic thought, for example, "I will be a laughing stock!"	Evidence for negative automatic thought, for example, "I feel that it might happen"	Evidence against negative automatic thought, for example, this has never happened before	New more balanced thought, for example, although I feel anxious nothing has happened in the past and is unlikely to happen this time	How does creating a new more balanced thought affect the way that I feel, e.g., anxiety reduces

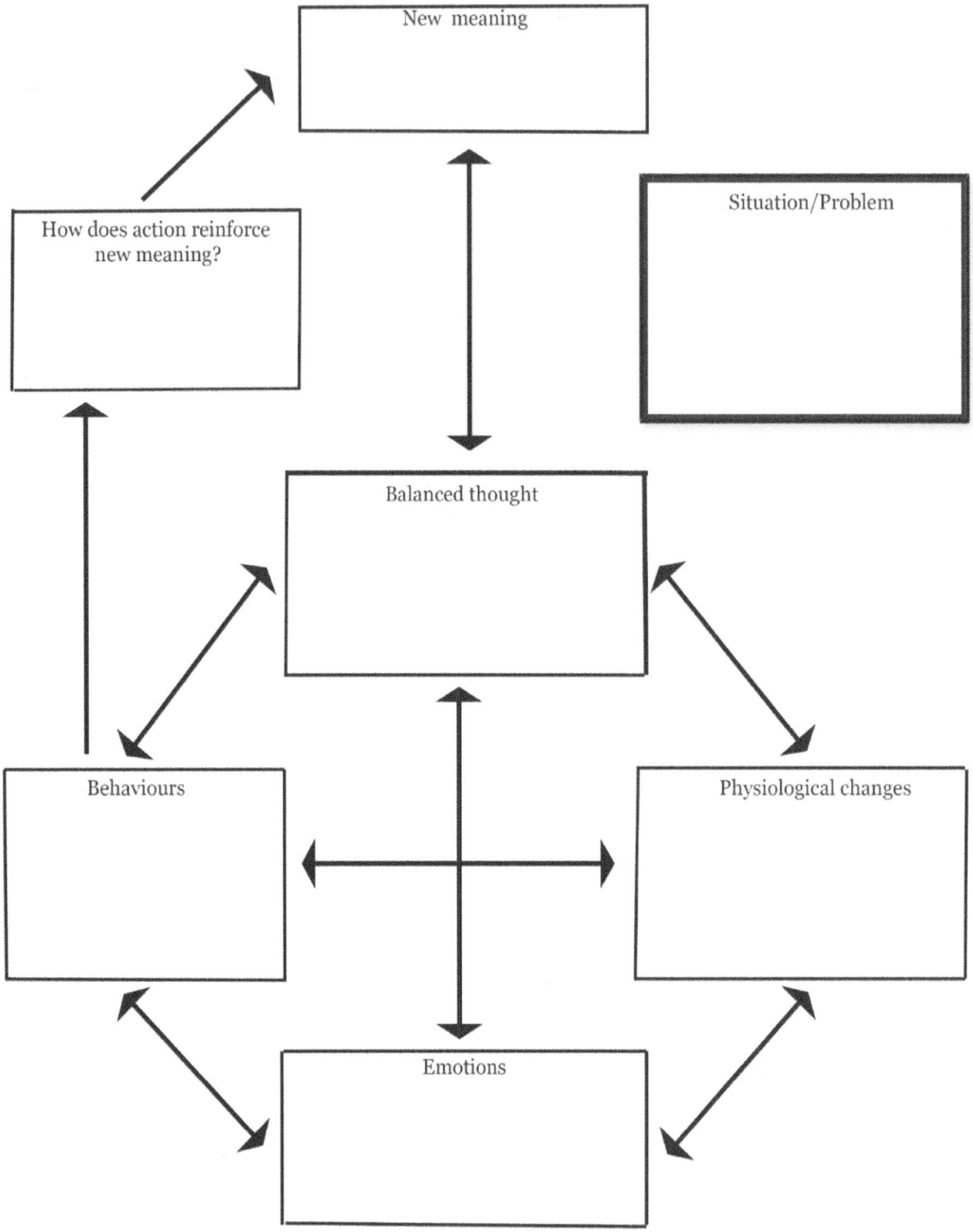

Figure 15. Positive maintenance cycle based on Christine Padesky's 'Hot-Cross Bun' approach

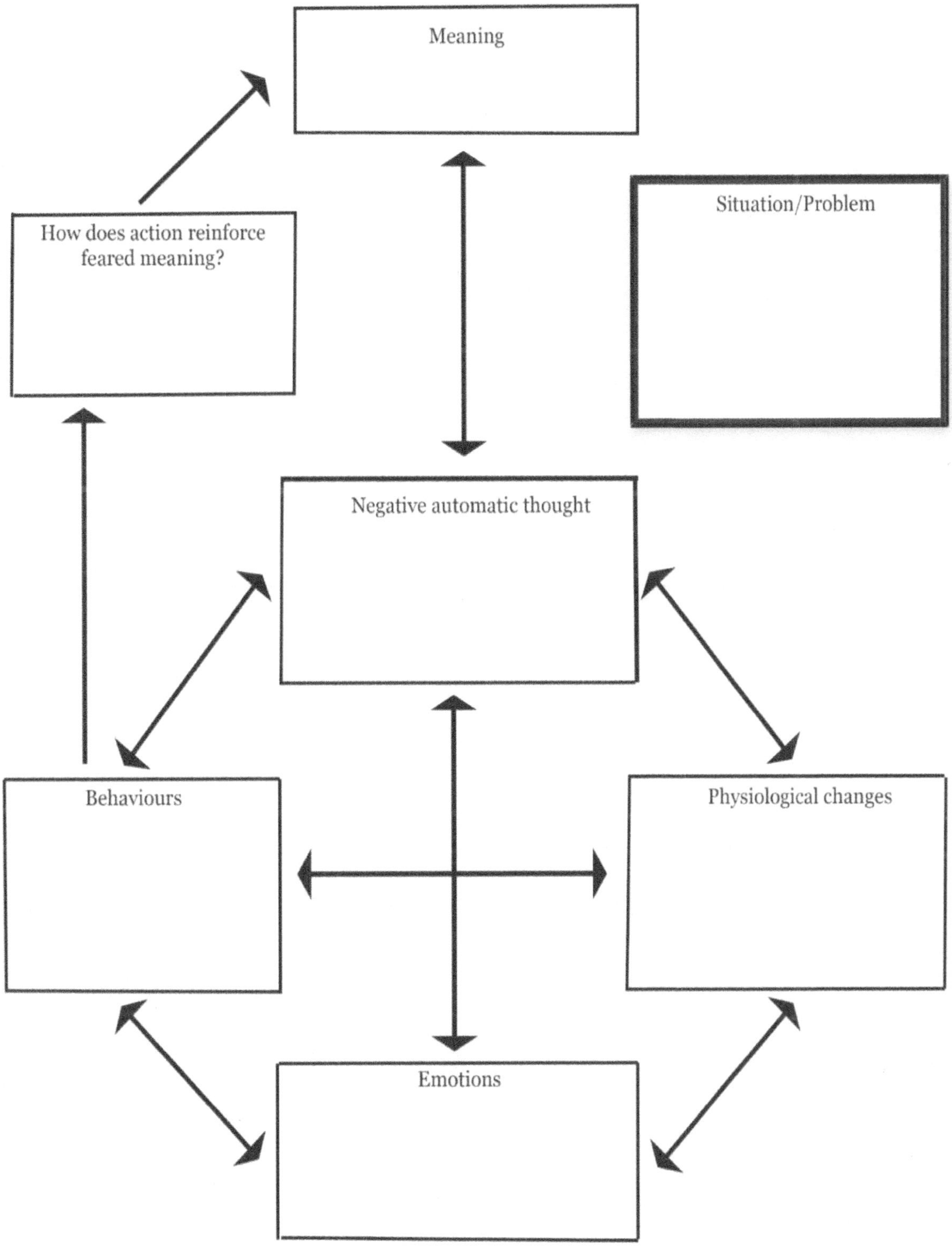

Figure 14. Negative maintenance cycle based on Christine Padesky's 'Hot-Cross Bun' approach

Table 11. NAT challenging form

Negative automatic thought, for example, "I will be a laughing stock!"	Evidence for negative automatic thought, for example, "I feel that it might happen"	Evidence against negative automatic thought, for example, this has never happened before	New more balanced thought, for example, although I feel anxious nothing has happened in the past and is unlikely to happen this time	How does creating a new more balanced thought affect the way that I feel, e.g., anxiety reduces

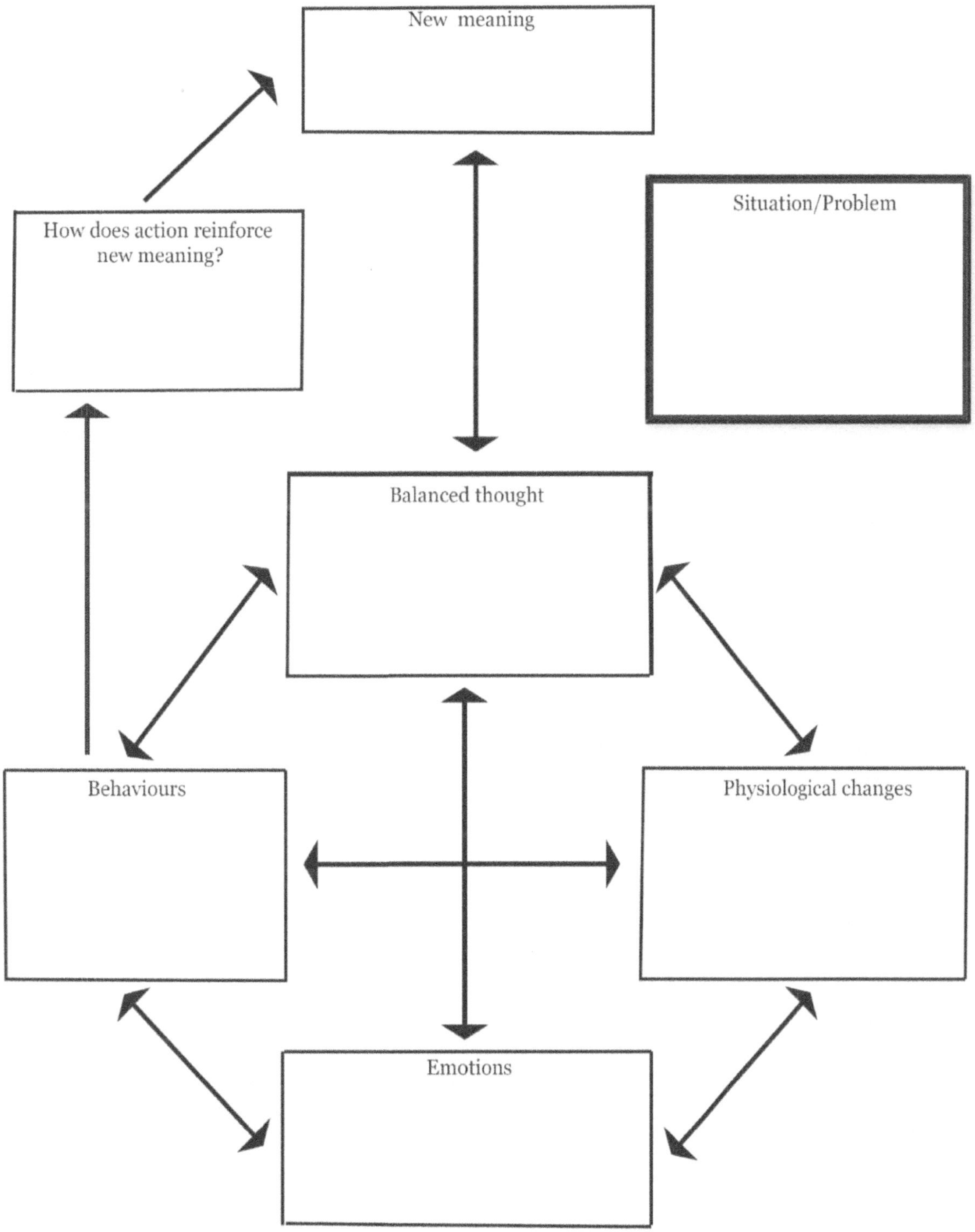

Figure 15. Positive maintenance cycle based on Christine Padesky's 'Hot-Cross Bun' approach

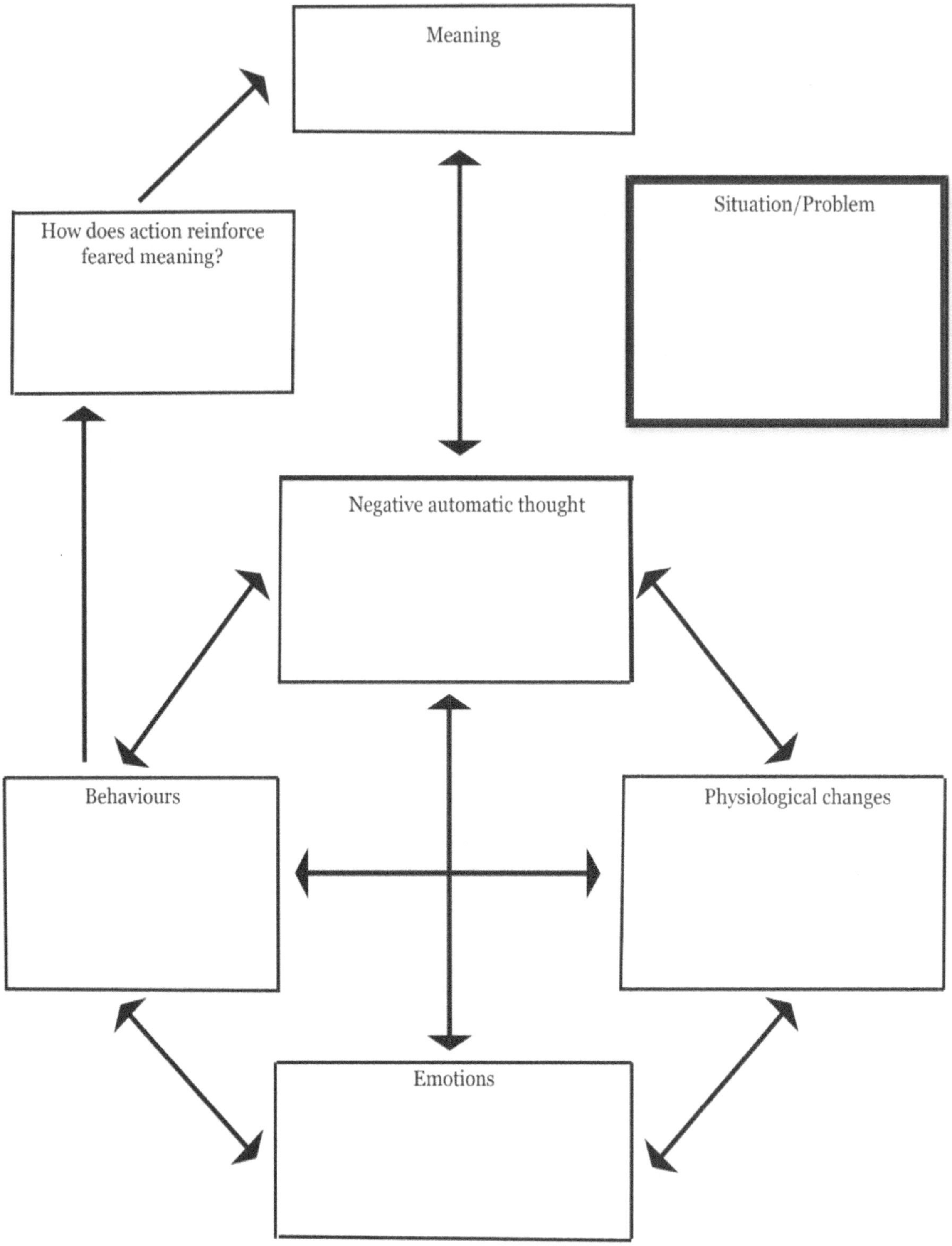

Figure 14. Negative maintenance cycle based on Christine Padesky's 'Hot-Cross Bun' approach

Table 11. NAT challenging form

Negative automatic thought, for example, "I will be a laughing stock!"	Evidence for negative automatic thought, for example, "I feel that it might happen"	Evidence against negative automatic thought, for example, this has never happened before	New more balanced thought, for example, although I feel anxious nothing has happened in the past and is unlikely to happen this time	How does creating a new more balanced thought affect the way that I feel, e.g., anxiety reduces

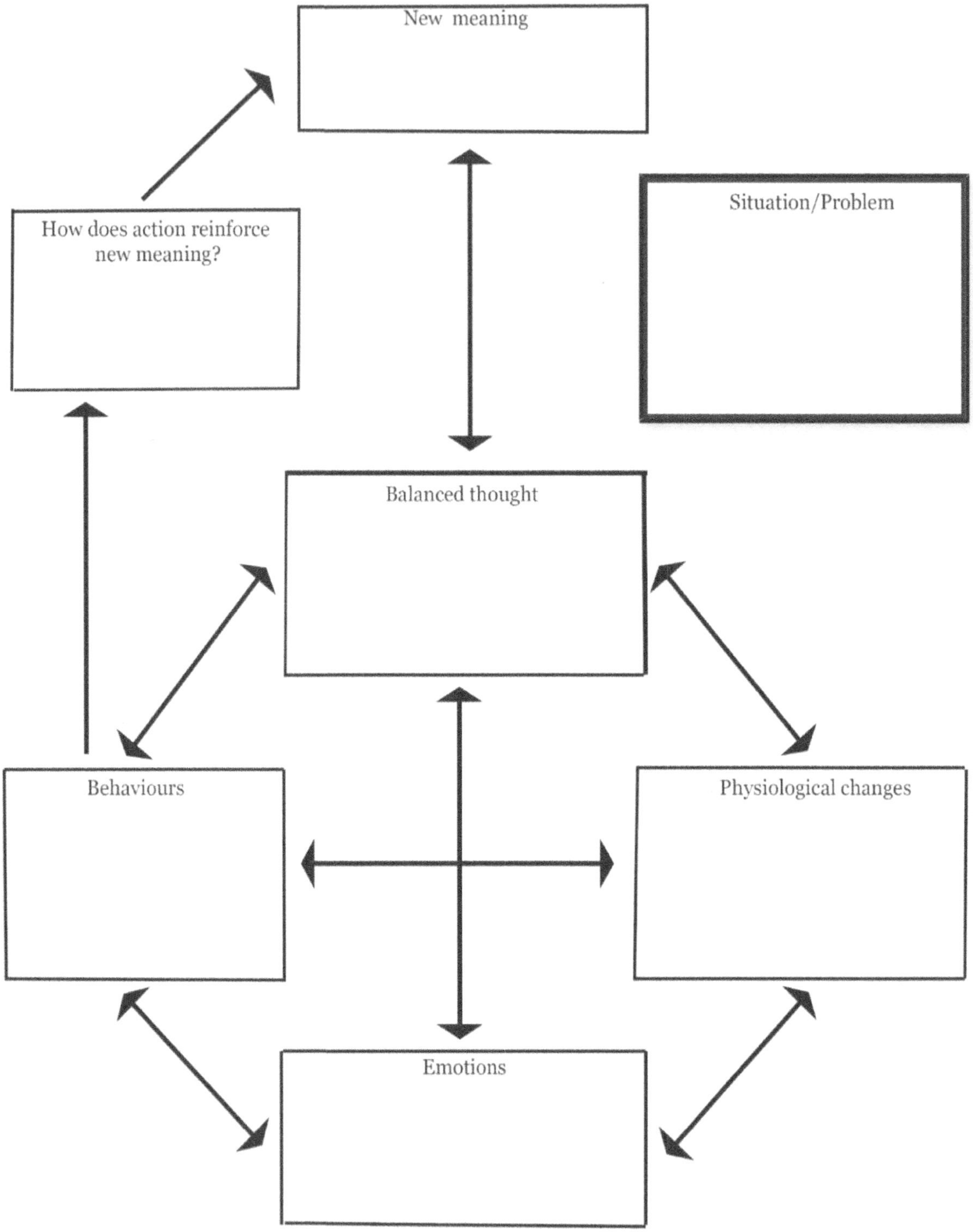

Figure 15. Positive maintenance cycle based on Christine Padesky's 'Hot-Cross Bun' approach

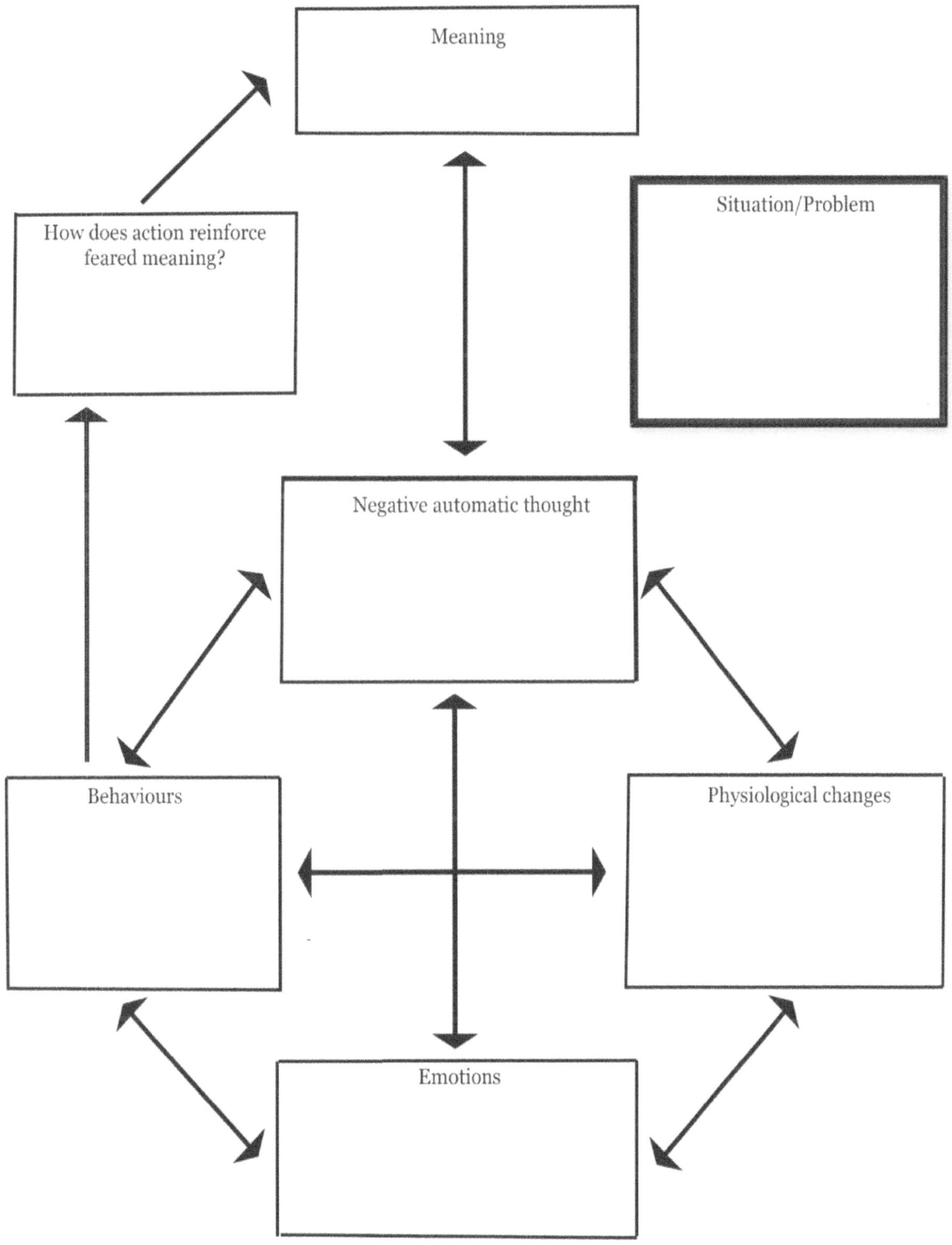

Figure 14. Negative maintenance cycle based on Christine Padesky's 'Hot-Cross Bun' approach

Table 11. NAT challenging form

Negative automatic thought, for example, "I will be a laughing stock!"	Evidence for negative automatic thought, for example, "I feel that it might happen"	Evidence against negative automatic thought, for example, this has never happened before	New more balanced thought, for example, although I feel anxious nothing has happened in the past and is unlikely to happen this time	How does creating a new more balanced thought affect the way that I feel, e.g., anxiety reduces

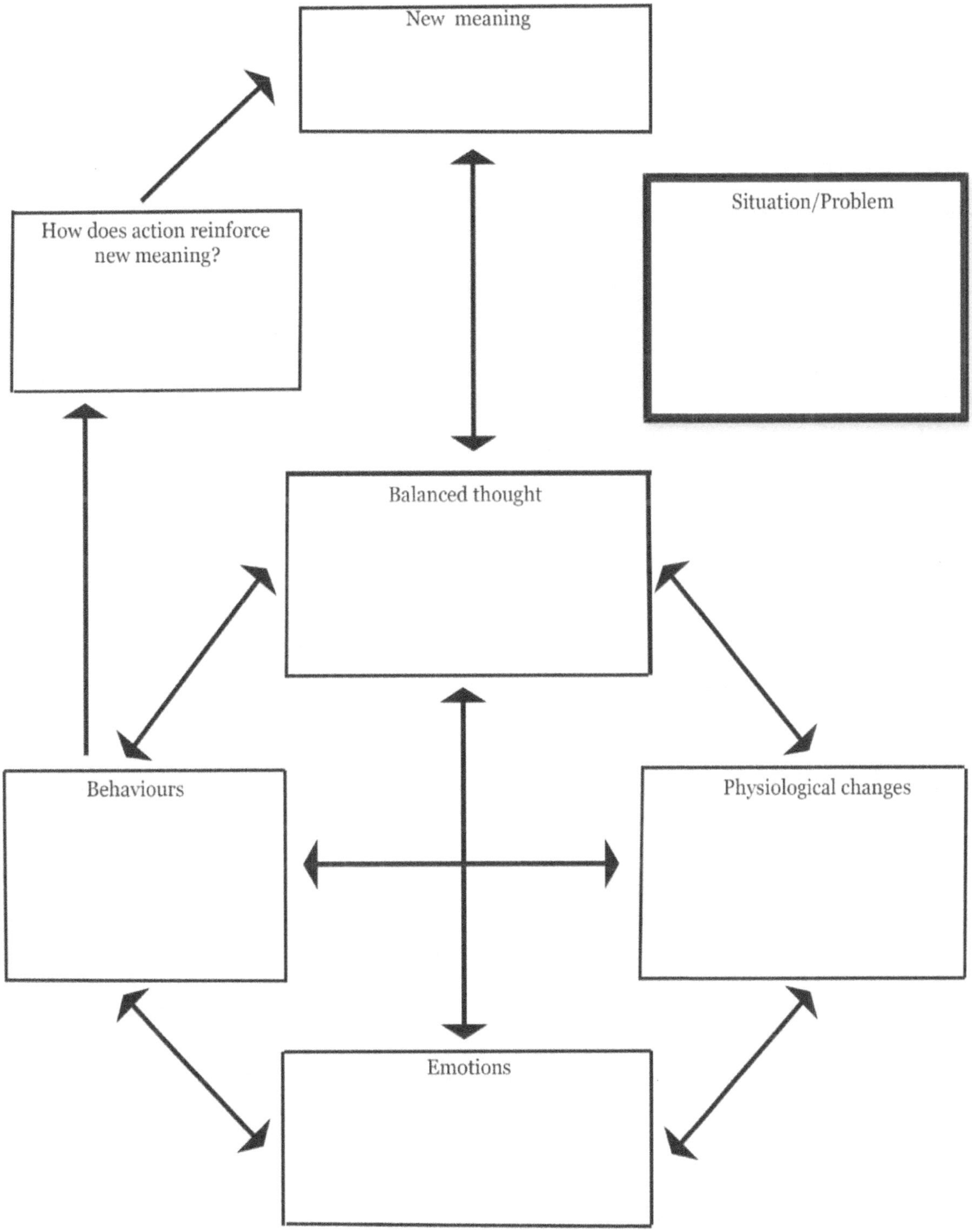

Figure 15. Positive maintenance cycle based on Christine Padesky's 'Hot-Cross Bun' approach

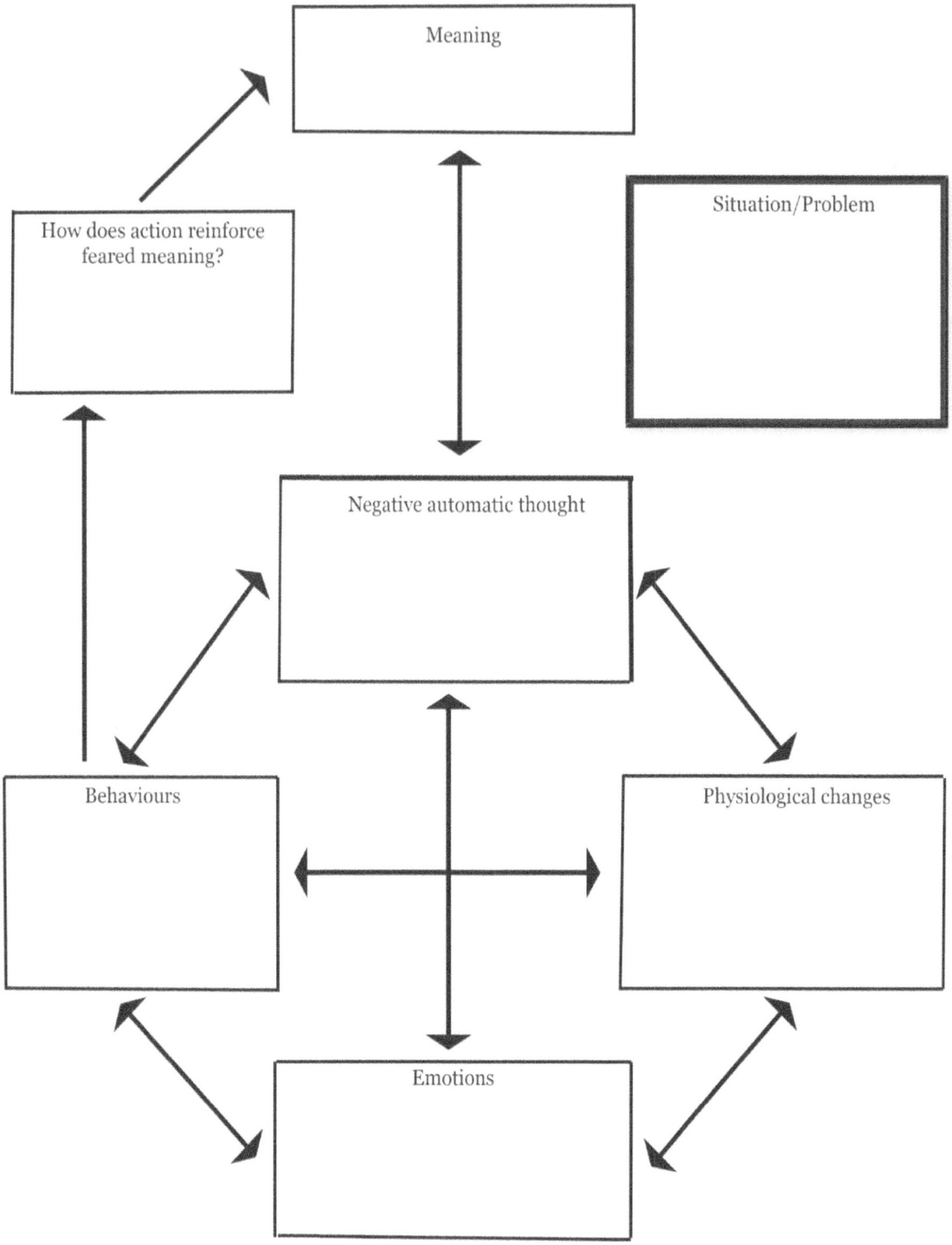

Figure 14. Negative maintenance cycle based on Christine Padesky's 'Hot-Cross Bun' approach

Table 11. NAT challenging form

Negative automatic thought, for example, "I will be a laughing stock!"	Evidence for negative automatic thought, for example, "I feel that it might happen"	Evidence against negative automatic thought, for example, this has never happened before	New more balanced thought, for example, although I feel anxious nothing has happened in the past and is unlikely to happen this time	How does creating a new more balanced thought affect the way that I feel, e.g., anxiety reduces

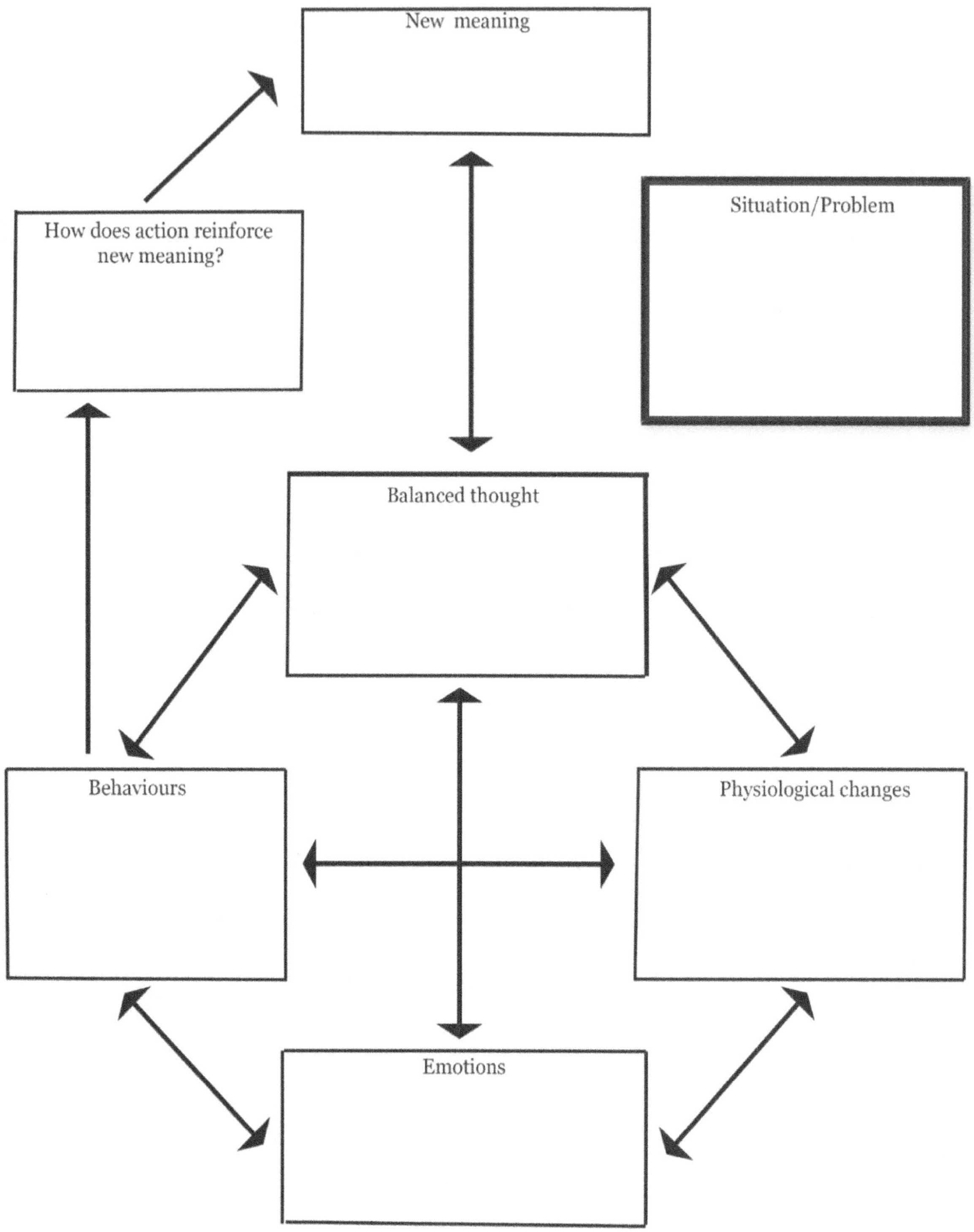

Figure 15. Positive maintenance cycle based on Christine Padesky's 'Hot-Cross Bun' approach

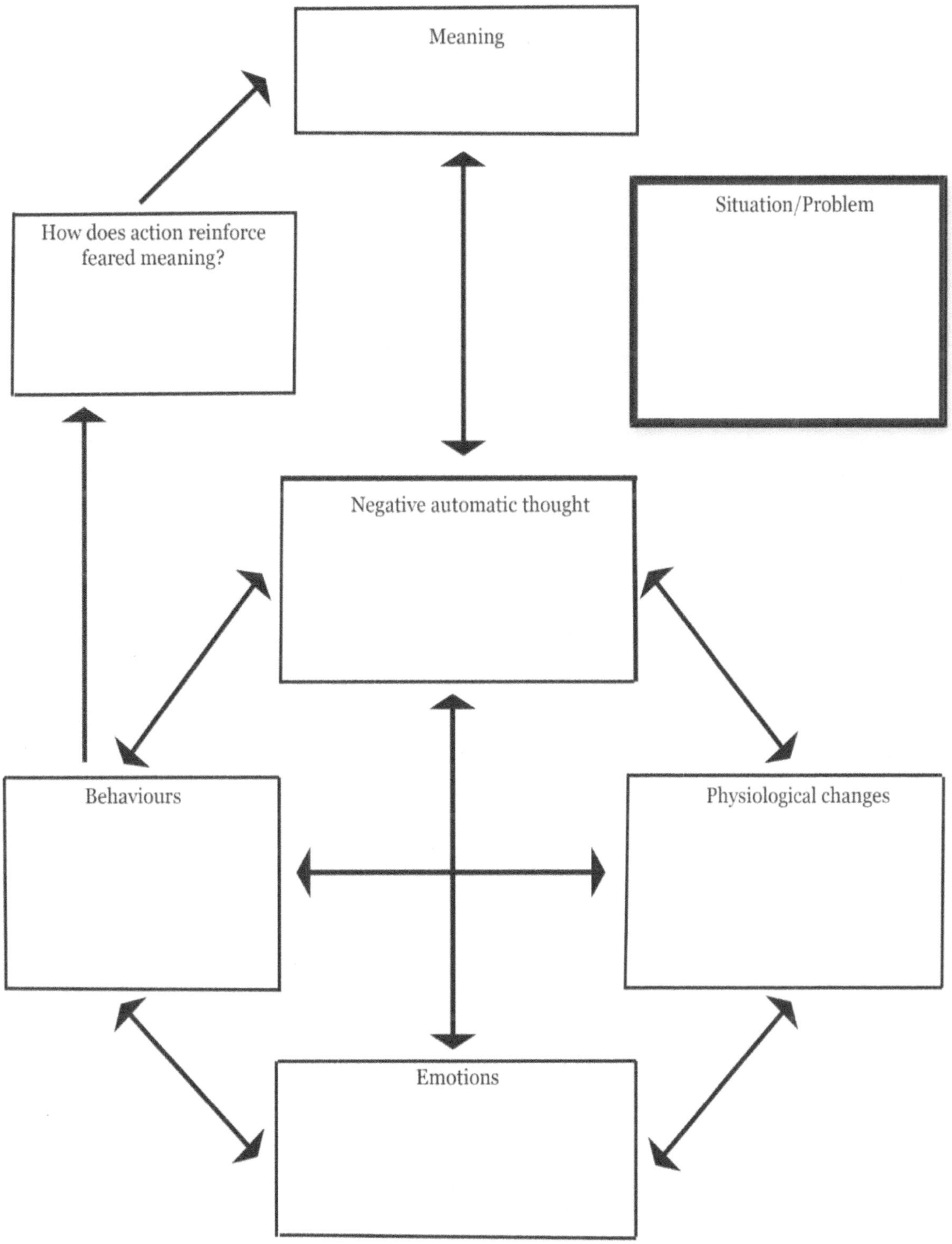

Figure 14. Negative maintenance cycle based on Christine Padesky's 'Hot-Cross Bun' approach

Table 11. NAT challenging form

Negative automatic thought, for example, "I will be a laughing stock!"	Evidence for negative automatic thought, for example, "I feel that it might happen"	Evidence against negative automatic thought, for example, this has never happened before	New more balanced thought, for example, although I feel anxious nothing has happened in the past and is unlikely to happen this time	How does creating a new more balanced thought affect the way that I feel, e.g., anxiety reduces

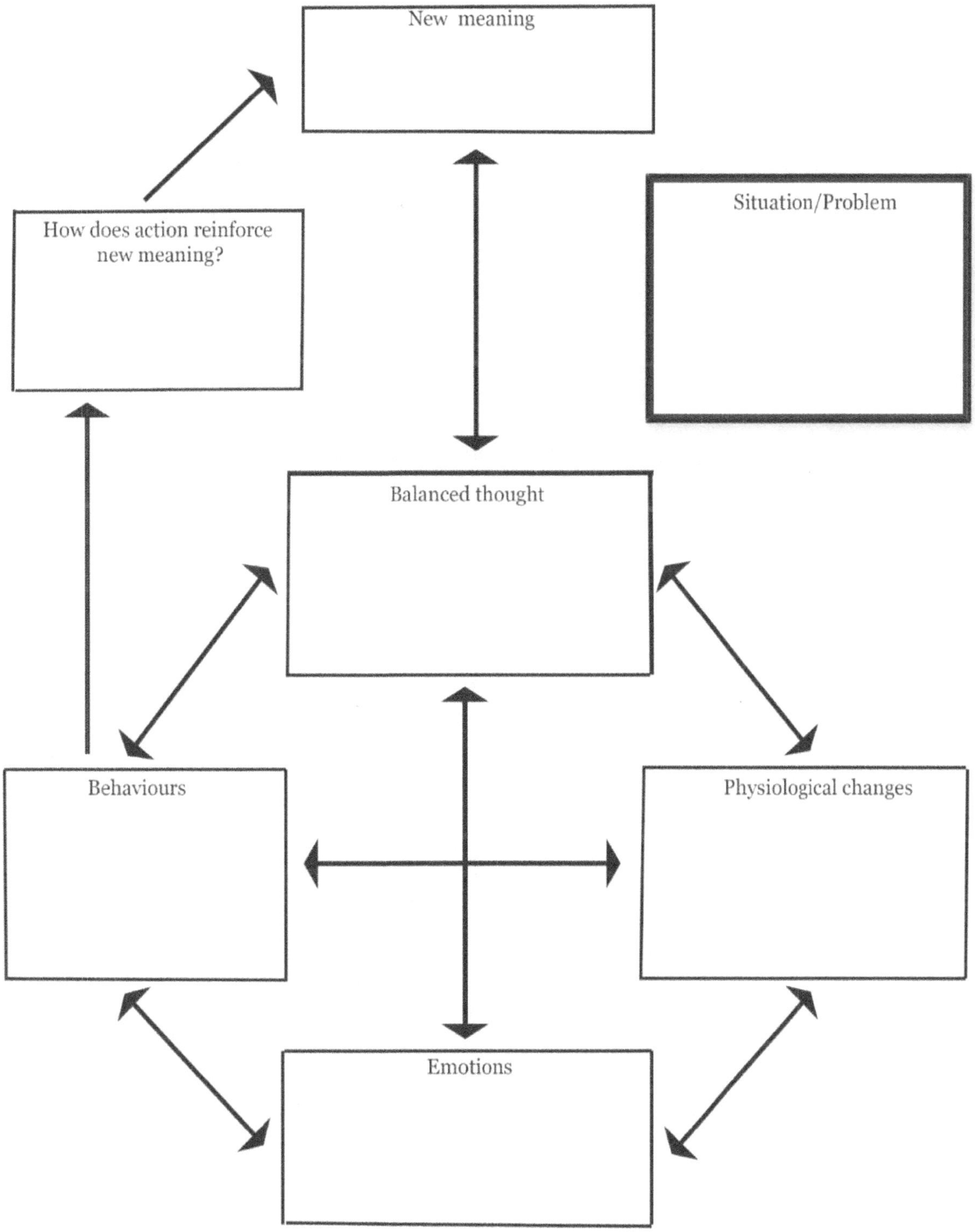

Figure 15. Positive maintenance cycle based on Christine Padesky's 'Hot-Cross Bun' approach

Chapter summary

Challenging NATs

- The first stage in challenging NATs is setting aside some time to notice the thoughts that are around when you feel very anxious.
- After you have noticed NATs you can just observe them and choose not to react to them, or you can challenge them.
- You can bring alternative explanations against your NATs to mind by using a thought challenging record.
- After you have completed a thought challenging record you can insert your new information into a positive CBT cycle.
- NATs have a habit of coming back so it is often very useful to get your thought challenging records out on a regular basis and spend some time re-reading them.

18 Approaching feelings

Melissa B, a teacher, was sitting in front of me. As she spoke she shifted around continuously in her chair, rubbing the back of her neck, grabbing her long red hair, breathing from the top of her chest, sighing and holding her breath at various times. She appeared to be a highly analytical person and was able to articulate her difficulties quite easily. She explained how interpersonal difficulties between herself and work colleagues had started, and she had insight into these problems. However, when I asked her how she was feeling in her body she found it extremely difficult to answer. It wasn't the case that Melissa didn't experience emotions as she was displaying them quite evidently in front of me through her body language. It was more simply a case that Melissa felt very uncomfortable when she recognised her bodily sensations of anxiety and felt a lot more familiar 'remaining or staying put in her head'. When I asked Melissa if she had ever developed any positive coping strategies to soothe herself she couldn't think of any. She stated quite simply that she had been brought up in a household where people didn't talk about their feelings. As a result of this from a very early age Melissa had naturally developed many sophisticated ways of ignoring or controlling her emotions and in fact had become quite an expert in emotional avoidance.

Figure 16. shows an example of the type of relationship that many individuals who experience social anxiety have with their feelings. Generally, painful emotions such as anxiety as well as anger and sadness are viewed as feelings to be feared or to be got rid of. As a result, strategies such as ignoring feelings, distracting the self from feeling feelings, and using safety behaviours to avoid feelings are commonly used. People's natural instinct is to supress uncomfortable feelings in order to feel better. However, an unfortunate consequence of engaging in emotionally avoidant strategies is that emotional distress is maintained at quite a high level or it increases even further over time.

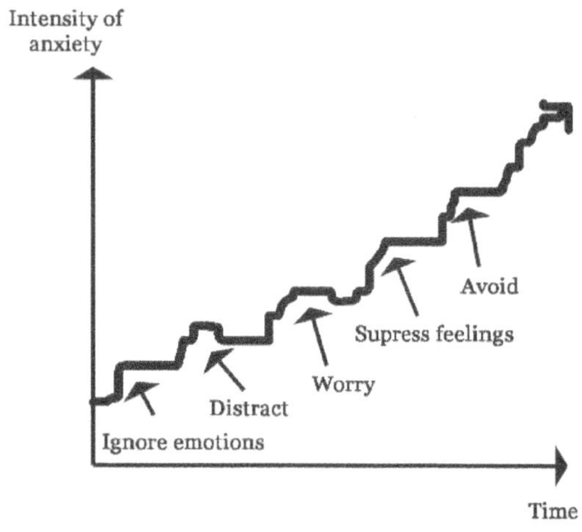

Figure 16. How people tend to react to their anxiety

A counter-intuitive solution to panic attacks and anxiety

The ideas covered in the right-hand column of the table on the next page (see table 12) often confuse my clients, because the concepts feel so alien to them. Maybe it's not dissimilar to asking them to grab a red-hot poker, while assuring them that it is not going to harm them. This type of '**counter-intuitive**' strategy to anxiety is the last thing that most people who experience anxiety would choose to do as they feel that their anxiety will rise significantly. By the way, when I say counter-intuitive I mean people carrying out behaviours or engaging in thoughts which are the direct opposite of what their intuition or feelings tell them is right.

In my sessions I ask my clients – "What would happen if you tried the opposite of what you normally do? For example, instead of ignoring emotions, you notice them and tell them that it is fine for them to be there?"

"What if instead of distracting yourself from anxiety, you focus on your feelings, and spend time in your body rather than in your head." I also ask – "What would happen if you begin to see anxiety as a friend rather than your enemy, if you allow your anxiety to be visible rather than try to hide it, and give permission for your anxiety to stay, rather than trying to get rid of it as soon as possible?"

Table 12. New strategy for feelings

Commonly applied solutions to anxiety	Strategy based on an opposite approach
Avoid uncomfortable feelings	Approach uncomfortable feelings
Distract self - Keep mind off of feelings	Focus on feelings
Perceive anxiety symptoms as threatening. Fear them	Perceive anxiety as part of the body that works for you. Embrace symptoms and allow symptoms to be visible
Control anxiety, try to get rid of feelings as soon as possible	Allow anxiety to freely move about body.
Tell anxiety that it shouldn't be there	Tell anxiety that that it OK to be there and that it can stay as long as it wants.

An effective wat to approach accepting feelings

If you remind yourself of the ideas covered in the early part of this book, you will remember that the neo-cortex is at the top of the brain, the prefrontal cortex is directly underneath that, and the sub-cortical regions are at the bottom of the brain. A slight problem for people who become highly anxious in social situations is that their pre-frontal cortex tends to go off-line when they are feeling most anxious. If this happens to you could find yourself in social situations, with your mind going blank, finding it very difficult to think clearly or rationally, and feeling unable to complete CBT exercises.

With this in mind, I suggest that a very useful starting point is to begin viewing yourself as a bit like a parent to the subcortical or primitive regions of the brain. Imagine these parts of the brain not as the enemy, but more like a servant that has worked for you loyally and tirelessly, a servant who is also very rarely appreciated for his or her effort.

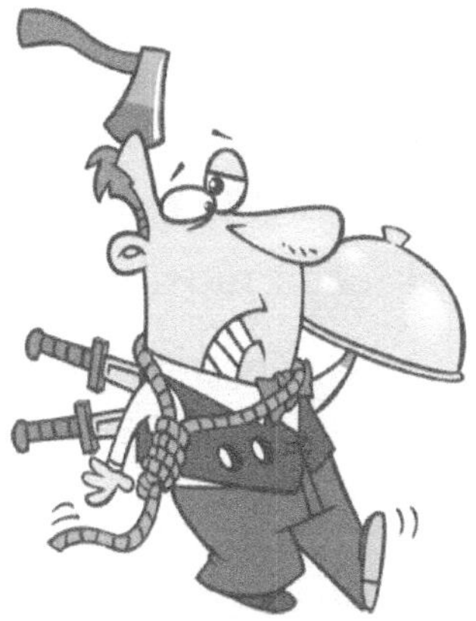

"I've got a niggling feeling that Madam's not very happy with me"

The best place to start your new parenting approach will be when you are on your own and when your anxiety levels are mild. Mild anxiety may be around, when you have day-to-day problems, for example, a problem at work, a problem with a friend or a relative etc. Mild distress may also be around when you worry, or when you ask "What if?" questions. The essence of the approach that I am going to suggest you use, is to become more aware of your feelings, especially anxious feelings at the earliest stage possible.

The best way to explain is with a demonstration. This is how a conversation with client might develop.

James: "OK, Jemma, I would just like you to think of a problem that you have had just recently, a problem that when you think about it now, still leaves you feeling slightly anxious."

Jemma: "OK, I've thought of something. Do you want me to talk to you about it?"

James: "No, I'd like you to keep it to yourself for now. I'd just like you to think about where you feel your emotions more strongly."

Jemma: "I feel it most in my chest!"

James: "Good. Keep your focus there. Now place one of your hands on your chest in the place where you feel your emotion more strongly. You are placing your hand on your body where your emotion is, because many of us who are prone to avoiding emotions unconsciously and automatically move away from feeling emotions, and go into our heads instead. You are gaining a connection with your emotions and keeping your focus on how you are feeling."

"Placing your hand on the part of your body where you feel your anxiety more strongly will also act as a reminder to you, to keep your focus on your emotions. It is very important while you are doing this exercise to focus on feeling your feelings and remind yourself that you really are willing for your emotions to be there."

"Focussing on the part of your body underneath you hand with your mind, examine exactly what your emotion feels like. For example, how much space do your feelings take up? How painful or uncomfortable are your feelings. Jemma, can you rate the intensity of your feeling between 1 and 10, where 10 is the highest level of intensity?"

Jemma: "They're about a 7 at the moment."

James: "OK, while you continue to feel your anxiety, mentally give it your permission to take up the space that it is taking up in your body. Taking things a little further I would also like you to speak internally with your anxiety saying something along the lines of the following."

"Thank you for being there" ... "There are very good reasons for you being there."

"Keep in mind the idea that from the primitive minds point of view there is a good reason for your anxiety being there, even if it does not make sense logically."

"Now follow that by saying "You are welcome to stay here for as long as you want."

"Bear in mind again Jemma from the primitive mind's point of view that if it notices during its screening process that there is a cue to a potential threat, which may be physical or psychological, it is just doing its job properly if it brings the threat to your attention and helps you to prepare.

The threat does not need to be valid in the current time mode. If it has been perceived as a threat in the past, or you have previously confirmed the existence of the threat by withdrawing from this threat in the past, then from the primitive mind's point of view the threat is still active."

"While feeling your symptoms of anxiety it is important when you speak to your feelings that you really mean what you are saying. Let go of all your thoughts and focus on your feeling. The importance of your self-communication is not in the words that you use but rather your intention behind your words. Keep an idea in mind of accepting, recognising, being grateful, and being patient. I'm just going to ask you to do this for a minute Jemma and we will see what happens."

...a minute passes...

James: "What are you noticing at the moment Jemma?"

Jemma: "The feeling is going down...It's about a 4 now."

James: "OK keep with the feeling, noticing that it is going down. Just stay with it. We'll see what happens in another minute or so."

...another minute passes...

James: "OK, Jemma what are you noticing now?"

Jemma: "It's gone!"

Learning how to stay with your feelings

I'd just like to complete a short recap now. It is important in the early stages of CBT that when you are experiencing anxiety, that you practice being with your feelings as much as possible. This will help you in two ways. Firstly, it will help you to fear your feelings less, and secondly it will make it more likely that you will be able to use your acceptance approach when you are experiencing higher levels of anxiety. You will need to bear in mind that in a state of heightened distress the frontal lobes - *where your self-soothing approach comes from* - stop working somewhat. Practicing acceptance over and over again when you are not so anxious will make it more likely that you will be able to access and use this self-soothing approach automatically when you need it.

The basal ganglia kicks in when we feel distressed

When we become highly anxious we are likely to continue to return to our old unhelpful habitual behaviours due to the strong influence of the basal ganglia which is located in the sub-cortical region of our brain. Activation of the basal ganglia results in us doing the same things that we have always done before. To change the use of unhelpful habits, you will need to practice using your new positive habits - learned through CBT exercises - over and over again. Eventually, your new CBT habits will come into place automatically when you are faced with distressing situations. This process takes time, however, as brain wiring in the basal ganglia does not grow instantly.

Teaching yourself how to reduce symptoms of social anxiety is determined by the relationship that you develop with yourself. Once high levels of anxiety are activated a cocktail of hormones is released into your blood stream and these hormones will need time to work their way through your system before you will be able to return to a more relaxed state.

Problems can occur if you react to fear in a critical, controlling or angry way. The primitive part of the self does not react well to being controlled, but it does react much more favourably to being noticed, to being thanked, to being treated non-judgementally, welcomed and soothed. In essence, a more adaptive strategy will be to move away from a controlling approach and move towards self-regulation and containment. Ostensibly, you will need to work on gaining the trust of the primitive part of the self. When that occurs the primitive part of the self will allow you to take charge.

Communicating with the primitive part of the self will involve listening and validating. If during a social situation you hear an internal voice stating that you are looking odd or weird it is important to hear what is being said, and to make a mental note of it.

Here follows a hypothetical communication between the neo-cortex and the primitive brain system.

Primitive brain – "I'm looking a bit awkward"

Neocortex – "What's happening?"

Primitive brain – "I'm feeling all tense"

Neocortex – "Yes, I am focusing on the feeling. I am noticing that your heart is beating faster, you're breathing faster, you're trembling a little and you feel really frightened"

Primitive brain – "I want to go"

Neocortex – "I understand that you want to get away"

Primitive brain – "Do something quickly, everyone is going to notice"

Neocortex – "You're really frightened at the moment, I know that feels really uncomfortable, these feelings are there because you're feeling anxious and you are worried others will notice. I am going to help you to focus on feeling these feelings and to help you to allow these uncomfortable feelings to be there. You will continue to feel frightened and very uncomfortable for a while because adrenaline is still pumping through your system. It will soon work its way through if you don't fight it. Allow yourself to breath more slowly and more deeply. It really is completely OK to feel anxious.

Primitive brain – "It's not so bad now"

The above dialogue may appear slightly artificial but it gives a sense of the type of compassionate communication that we are aiming for. To reduce your symptoms of social anxiety you will need to train your neo-cortex to be compassionate, to listen, to validate, and to form a positive relationship with the primitive part.

Chapter summary
Approaching feelings

- Most individuals who experience social anxiety tend to remain in analytical mode.
- Avoiding feeling emotions tends to keep fear in place and prolongs suffering.
- Counter-intuitive approaches such as focussing on uncomfortable feelings, making room for feelings, and validating anxiety produce positive results in the long-term.
- A useful strategy is to form a positive relationship with the primitive part of the mind.
- The primitive part of the mind has valid reasons for reacting to psychological and physiological threats and is working to protect you, not to harm you. Its intention is to help!

Chapter 18 - Homework

Using the record sheet (see table 13) keep a record of your anxiety level before and after you practice making room for your feelings. What do you predict will occur?

Table 13. Accepting emotions record

Use this worksheet to keep a record of your anxiety level before and after you practice making room for your feelings. What do you predict will occur?				
Date/Time	**Trigger**	**Anxiety level before accepting feelings between 0 and 10 (where 10 is the highest it can be)**	**Anxiety level after completing exercise**	**Observations while completing the exercise**

Table 13. Accepting emotions record

Use this worksheet to keep a record of your anxiety level before and after you practice making room for your feelings. What do you predict will occur?

Date/Time	Trigger	Anxiety level before accepting feelings between 0 and 10 (where 10 is the highest it can be)	Anxiety level after completing exercise	Observations while completing the exercise

Table 13. Accepting emotions record

Use this worksheet to keep a record of your anxiety level before and after you practice making room for your feelings. What do you predict will occur?				
Date/Time	**Trigger**	**Anxiety level before accepting feelings between 0 and 10 (where 10 is the highest it can be)**	**Anxiety level after completing exercise**	**Observations while completing the exercise**

Table 13. Accepting emotions record

Use this worksheet to keep a record of your anxiety level before and after you practice making room for your feelings. What do you predict will occur?

Date/Time	**Trigger**	**Anxiety level before accepting feelings between 0 and 10 (where 10 is the highest it can be)**	**Anxiety level after completing exercise**	**Observations while completing the exercise**

19 How worry and rumination make things worse

Most people who experience social anxiety will spend a significant portion of their time worrying or ruminating. Because these processes tend to maintain emotional difficulties it is important that we take a look at them.

Rumination is a process of churning negative thoughts over in one's mind. Most ruminative thoughts are connected to the self and the past. Some people suggest that rumination is useful because it can help to create lots of possibilities, and can offer solutions when we are faced with specific problems.

Rumination, however, does not work well when we try to analyse our way out of emotional distress.

A process of rumination is kept in place by the questions we ask ourselves. For example, if we ask "Why does this keep happening to me" or "What's wrong with me?" The questions that we ask ourselves throw up answers which, in turn, can lead us to ask more questions. Before long, if this process continues unstopped we can end up confirming our worst fears, for example, that we are worthless, wrong, useless, bad, and such like. The irony of the whole process is that in our search for ways to avoid current or future painful feelings by ruminating, we end up dwelling on the past and we can end up feeling worse than ever. It's not dissimilar to using a shovel to dig ourselves out of a hole. The more we dig, the deeper the hole gets! The problem is that often we do not feel that we have any other way of solving our problems, so we continue to use the same strategy, even though we know it does not work. I'll just give a hypothetical example now about how a conversation might go between a CBT therapist and a client.

CLIENT - "What's the difference between worry and rumination?"

CBT THERAPIST - "Worry and rumination are similar in that they both involve thought churning. The main difference between them is that worry is focussed on the future and being able to cope with potential outcomes, whereas rumination is focussed on the past."

"When people worry they think about upcoming situations and ask questions such as "What will I do if this happens?" "What is the worst thing that could happen?" or "What if this happens?" They do this because they think that if they can imagine the worst case scenario, then they will be able to put things in place to deal with whatever happens in a particular situation. They think if they can work out what might happen in advance then they will be safe. Ironically, however, just like rumination, in an attempt to achieve certainty and to feel safe, we can end up feeling more frightened than ever, and also experience intrusive thoughts."

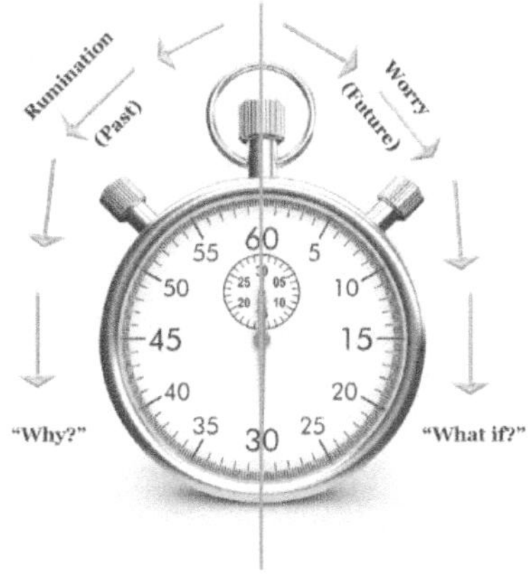

CLIENT - "Intrusive thoughts?"

CBT THERAPIST – "An intrusive thought is a thought that pushes its way into awareness with extreme urgency. Intrusive thoughts often appear to come out of nowhere and carry high levels of emotional distress with them. Ironically, intrusive thoughts alone can trigger high levels of anxiety."

"Before I explain why intrusive thoughts may occur, I want to offer you a simple analogy about the functioning of the mind."

"First I'd like you to recognise that they have a **conscious mind.** When people use their conscious minds they are awake to thoughts, images or sensations that they experience. I'd like us to imagine that the conscious mind is a bit like a magic white board that begins to erase what is written on it after only a few seconds. Because the ink or information expressed using the ink disappears so rapidly the only way to keep anything live on this white board is to continuously write on it over and over again. When new information is written on the white board, information that was on the white board previously, disappears even more rapidly. A further point to note is that the amount of information that can be written on the whiteboard at any one point in time is limited due to the whiteboards small size."

CLIENT - "So you saying the mind is like a white-board. I'm not sure I understand?"

CBT THERAPIST - "Do you mind if I demonstrate with you? It's much easier to show you how this works rather than to explain it. Before we start I just want to let you know that this is not a test. It's just a little exercise so that you can find out how much information your mind can hold onto. I am going to start by asking you to remember five random numbers and letters. Are you ready?

CLIENT - "Yes"

CBT THERAPIST - "5A3KQ. Have you got that?"

CLIENT - "Yes. I think so!"

CBT THERAPIST – "Alright I now want you to remember these numbers as well."

"27KR1...Right, can you repeat that sequence for me?"

CLIENT - "27KR1"

CBT THERAPIST - "Good...And, the first sequence"

CLIENT - "...Erm ... [a big pause follows] ...57...Q...It seems to have gone out of my head... I'm sorry."

CBT THERAPIST - "There's no need to be sorry. This is exactly what is meant to happen. This is how the mind works. We just gave your internal whiteboard an impossible task. Hardly anyone can recall over 9 randomly presented units of information unless they use specialised memory techniques, and I just gave you 10. That's why I'm saying the whiteboard is small."

"I'll just explain it a bit more. A benefit of the white board's disappearing ink process is that it is constantly available for continuous use. As a result of this, huge amounts of information can be written on the whiteboard during the period of its lifetime. In many respects, it could be suggested that we could feel grateful that the whiteboard loses access to information so quickly. If it didn't it would quite quickly become jammed up with too much information and become unusable."

"Taking this idea further, I'd like us to imagine that our **out of conscious processes** work a little bit like a building that the white board is housed in. I'll just explain that out of conscious processes are brain functions that we are unaware of, or mental processes that go on in the back of our minds."

CLIENT - "And, what's the significance of associating the out of conscious mind with a building?"

CBT THERAPIST - "I'm saying that out of conscious processes are like a building because the amount of brain space required for out of conscious thinking is absolutely huge in in comparison to the amount of brain used for the white board. The building is also three dimensional unlike the two dimensional whiteboard, there are also multiple rooms, and secret passageways.

CLIENT - "I understand why it is big but what does the three dimensional layout of the building represent, with multiple rooms and such like?"

CBT THERAPIST - "This represents an idea that the out of conscious mind can think on several different levels at the same time. It can absorb information from our environment, take care of all of our bodily functions, plan our activities, assist our communication, and think about problems we have in our lives without us being aware of it. It can also use symbols, images, and words to create ideas and connect them up in a way that we would struggle to do consciously. What it can do is really quite incredible!"

"In this building there are also filing cabinets crammed with information that we thought we had forgotten about, and there are reams of papers lying around waiting to be filed."

CLIENT - "What do the reams of papers represent?"

CBT THERAPIST - "The reams of paper represent thoughts that we have not fully processed or ideas that we are currently working on. Many people may have several hundred or even thousands of different thoughts strands they are working on at any one time. Thought strands may be about relationships with different people, hobbies or interests, work projects, holidays and such like. Information does not disappear easily from this building but very often it can get lost or misfiled."

CLIENT - "So how does it get lost or misfiled?"

CBT THERAPIST - "There is so much information in this building or in peoples' minds that sometimes it is hard for them to find what they are looking for. The more information that's in the building the harder it is to find what they need."

"Now imagine that in this building there is a little librarian who is very loyal to you and will try to find answers to anything that you ask using the whiteboard, even if it means working through the night. Sometimes the librarian finds information quickly, sometimes it might take days, but when the librarian finds answers to questions posed on the whiteboard it will post it an answer on the whiteboard just as soon as space becomes available."

CLIENT - "I'm still not sure I still fully understand this analogy of a librarian. How does this work with real problems?"

CBT THERAPIST - "OK. Let's imagine that you are walking down the street one day and on the other side of the street there is a girl whose face you recognise. You are immediately aware that you know her but this is not where you usually see her. You ask yourself "Where do I know her from?" a few times. Nothing comes to her mind immediately and you carry on doing whatever you were doing before. You may even forget that you asked that question as it disappears from your conscious awareness and it is replaced by other things. However, a little while later, maybe a few hours, days, or sometimes weeks later, an idea pops into your mind telling you where you knew the person you saw in the street from. How do you think this might happen?"

CLIENT - "Well I guess the little librarian had not forgotten that I asked that question, perhaps she was going through the filing cabinets looking for an answer or maybe she waited for me to go somewhere and suddenly remembered."

CBT THERAPIST - "That's what I'm saying. As soon as an opportunity occurred and there was space available on the whiteboard the librarian posted the information. A useful rule of thumb, therefore, will be to assume that when we ask our brain a question it will continue to work on questions posed to it even though we may have consciously forgotten that we have asked the questions in the first place."

"Usually the little librarian will put thoughts or information in a queue to enter conscious awareness, and in this respect answers to questions you have asked will wait patiently to pop into your mind when there is space available or when the mind is not occupied with something else."

CLIENT - "Is that why so many thoughts go through my head at night just as I want to go to sleep?"

CBT THERAPIST - "Yes, that what I'm getting at. You will have access to these thoughts at night because your mind is not focussed on other things.

CLIENT - "What about the other thoughts you mentioned earlier. I think you said they were intrusive thoughts. I used to get those a lot?"

CBT THERAPIST - "Intrusive thoughts are different to the above mentioned patient type of thoughts that we have. They are not dissimilar to the librarian pushing through a registered letter for your attention. Intrusive thoughts are pushed through to consciousness, as a priority, pushing out any other information that is currently on line. You may be talking with someone when one of these thoughts pops into your head. For example, an image of yourself looking odd could suddenly be pushed into your mind. Intrusive thoughts are sent with high degrees of importance and you will notice them as a result of the emotional intensity that comes with them."

CLIENT - "So where do they come from?"

CBT THERAPIST – "There may be many factors responsible for the creation of intrusive thoughts. One way that they may be generated is by worrying or asking "What if?" questions. This type of questioning process certainly appears to increase the likelihood of intrusive thoughts being pushed into consciousness. It is important to recognise than that when we receive intrusive thought messages they are not 'evidence' for anything. Although intrusive thoughts often feel uncomfortable, because they bring fear with them, it does not make these thoughts any more real than any other thoughts that pop into your mind."

"I think the best way to explain this is by talking about a young man I worked with a little while ago."

"Gregory was a big worrier. He would often go through a process of worry, asking "What if?" questions to his mind and his brain would usually send him back the worst possible things that could happen, or what could go wrong. His intentions for worrying were positive as he felt that this type of questioning process could keep him safe. He thought that if he knew about the types of problems that might occur in advance then he could be prepared for them. Before going to the cinema with friends Gregory would ask himself about what could go wrong. His obedient mind usually sent him answers. One type of answer generated and sent to his conscious awareness was that he may end up in a middle seat feeling panicky, with everyone around noticing him, and he would feel humiliated."

CLIENT - "I think most people would be anxious about that, wouldn't they?"

CBT THERAPIST - "They might do if they worried a lot about what people thought about them. But remember nothing had *actually* happened at this point. This was all in his mind. But, based on the ideas that his mind gave him Gregory decided to take action and sit at the back near an aisle seat so that he could make a quick exit if required. Gregory then began to think of how he could position himself in an aisle seat. He thought that if he could go in first in his group of friends he could stand near an aisle seat and gesture to others to go in ahead of him. His mind came up with a further ideas, such as if anyone questioned his need to sit in an aisle seat, he would say that he had a stomach ache and may need to go to the bathroom. He also had thoughts about phoning his friends up at the last minute and telling them that he couldn't make it. The amount of worrying that Gregory experienced before going to the cinema made the whole process of going to the cinema a difficult experience rather than the enjoyable experience that it could have been. Gregory's mind also reminded him how strange he was for engaging in this type of behaviour, and his friends would never think that he was like that."

CLIENT - "So what happened to him?"

CBT THERAPIST - "A big risk for Gregory was deciding not to ask "What if?" questions. A big part of Gregory thought that asking himself these questions kept him prepared, safe and not vulnerable. Recognising that all thoughts that come into awareness are simply offerings sent by the mind and not ideas supported by evidence made a significant difference to Gregory. Gregory learnt how to stand back and observe his thoughts, and recognise that any thought that came into awareness was just a suggestion. Just because he had a thought did not mean it needed to be dealt with. As such, learning to notice his thoughts made a significant difference to him."

"Many people's minds come up with all sorts of negative ideas when they worry. In Gregory's case a worry for him was losing control, being thought of by others as weak, and others thinking that there was something wrong with him. I drew a diagram on my office whiteboard for Gregory to look at. I have copied this onto the next page. It's similar to the diagrams that Christine Padesky uses."

CLIENT - "Isn't she one of the authors of the book 'Mind over Mood?"

CBT THERAPIST - "That right! Christine Padesky's ideas are very useful to us here to explain what was happening to Gregory. Gregory engaged in numerous avoidant type behaviours which tended to confirm his fear based thoughts still further. By carrying out avoidant behaviours Gregory did not collect alternative evidence that challenged his fears."

CBT THERAPIST - "Gregory's example shows how the interactions between thoughts, feelings and behaviour have a tendency to maintain problems. In this case, interfering with Gregory's worry processes led to him having less frightening thoughts, which in turn led to a reduction in his tendency to want to avoid situations."

Research

Intrusive thoughts are defined as unwanted thoughts images or impulses. In 2014 Richard Moulding & his colleagues completed an international study to identify a) the prevalence of intrusive thoughts and b) how people react to them. They assessed 777 students across 15 cities, 13 countries, and 6 continents. They found that 93 percent of their students experienced intrusive thoughts in the previous 3 months, suggesting that intrusive thoughts are in fact a normal part of daily living. The researchers' natural conclusion was therefore - It is not the intrusive thoughts themselves that maintain mental health problems, but rather it is how we react to them.

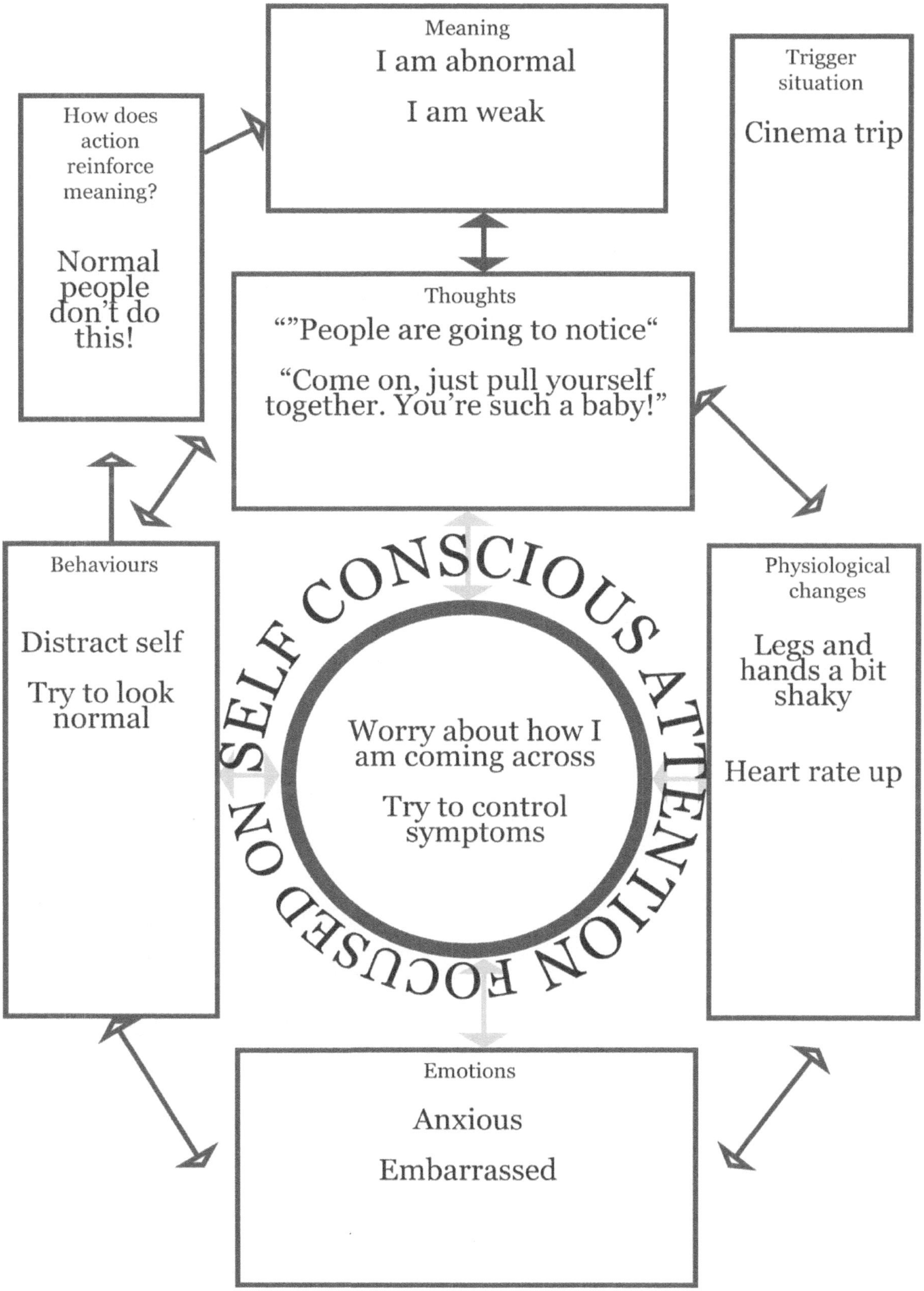

Figure 17. Social anxiety cycle

Chapter summary

How worry and rumination make things worse

- Worry does not happen by itself. It is a safety mechanism that many of us use to help us feel prepared for upcoming situations.

- The frequency of intrusive thoughts during social events are increased by the worry process.

- Intrusive thoughts, although frightening are no more fact-based that any other thought.

- The emotional impact of thoughts can be reduced by noticing them rather than reacting to them.

- Avoiding situations as a result of believing intrusive thoughts can lead to problems being maintained.

20

Retraining the sub-cortical mind

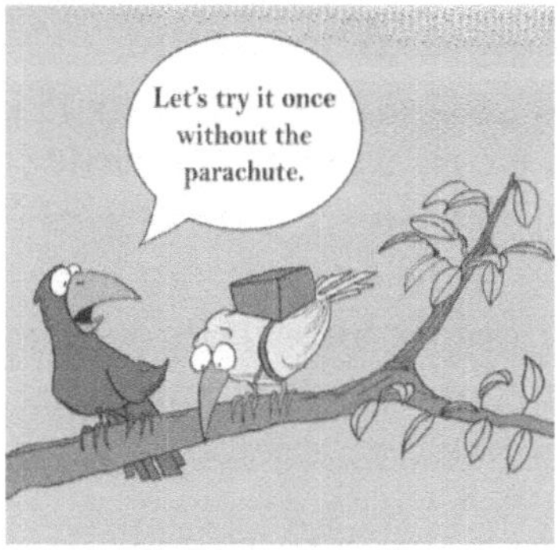

As many of us are aware, when we worry about the potential outcomes of social experiences, reassuring ourselves appears to have a limited impact. You may well have read the contents of this book and hopefully by now have more knowledge about social anxiety. However, despite this you may continue to experience intense feelings of anxiety in social situations. If you are at this stage, your neocortex understands how social anxiety maintains itself, but the primitive part of your brain has yet to take on board the same information.

With this in mind one of the most helpful ways to teach the primitive mind how to absorb new information is through experience. I will explain using an analogy.

I would like to invite you to think of the primitive mind as a child who comes to your bedroom door one night feeling frightened. You ask the child what she is frightened of and she says that she thinks there is something – a monster - in her wardrobe. You have several options in terms of your response.

- You could tell the child not to be so silly and completely ignore her. The result of this is that that the child waits around outside your room and continues to try to gain your attention. She could even wait outside your bedroom door for the whole night.
- You could rationalise with the child. You explain to her how impossible it is that a monster could get into her wardrobe and that monsters don't exist. You tell her that she is thinking about monsters because she watched a frightening television programme about monsters earlier. The result of this is that the child nods while listening and goes back to her room for a short while, but is back outside your room a few minutes later.
- You could tell the child that she can sleep in a put-down bed in your room. The child is not scared anymore and happily gets into this bed. However, when the next day comes she seems more terrified than before of sleeping in her bedroom.

Or

- You could take the child's hand acknowledging that she feels really frightened and tell her that you are both going to look into the wardrobe together. When you approach the wardrobe the child is really scared and she tries to resist going towards the wardrobe. You gently persist telling the child that it really is OK to feel frightened. When you have opened the wardrobe door and you both have had a good look inside for a couple of minutes you notice that the child has become a lot less anxious and is happier once more to sleep in her own bed. You don't hear any more from the child until you see her the next morning.

With the fourth option you don't have to explain or rationalise, you simply help the child to acknowledge that she is scared. You take her to the situation which you know logically is very low risk (i.e., there is a very low probability of there being a monster in her wardrobe) and encourage her to find out for herself how dangerous the situation is. The child learns by her own experience.

There is one more thing to note in this area. The child looking in the wardrobe will need to do this without carrying out any ritualistic behaviours or safety mechanisms. These could include crossing fingers, closing her eyes, holding onto a teddy bear etc. If the child uses these things for reassurance then the child will believe that her safety behaviours are keeping her safe and she will continue to need them. Remember many people who experience panic attacks have safety behaviours, such as carrying diazepam, using beta-blockers, worrying, distracting the self by listening to music etc.

In the next chapter we will look at eliminating safety behaviours using a route of least resistance.

Chapter summary

Retraining the sub-cortical mind

- The subcortical mind does not update itself automatically as you acquire new knowledge

- The subcortical mind learns through direct experience. It needs to be shown that things are OK, rather than be told that things are OK.

21

Behavioural experiments with social anxiety

Behavioural experiments can be very helpful in challenging the behaviours that maintain social anxiety. The general idea behind them is to teach the self to learn positive behaviour change through breaking patterns of old unhelpful behaviour. To carry out a behavioural experiment you will need to make a decision to change a behaviour and then put yourself directly in a position to make that behaviour change happen. You will need to make a prediction before the behaviour is carried out, (what you think or feel might happen). When you carry out your new behaviour it is important that you record the results. The majority of us make assumptions about a) how others might react to our behaviour, or b) how we might feel if we carry out a certain behaviour. A lot of the time, however, our assumptions are based on inaccurate information or indeed a lack of knowledge. Behavioural experiments help with the development of experiential knowledge.

In my clinical practice I regularly carry out behavioural experiments with my clients. Typically, behavioural experiments can be used to challenge safety behaviours used to cope in social situations, such as focusing on the self, monitoring the self for signs of anxiety and such like. I have placed a number of potential behavioural experiments over the next few pages for you to take a look at (see tables 14a to 14d).

Completing a behavioural experiment will involve you making a prediction about what you think may occur if you change your behaviour in a particular situation. After you have made a prediction, you will then carry out your new behaviour and observe what occurs. I have created some tables to help you with this (see table 15.)

Table 14a. Potential behavioural experiments for social anxiety

Current behaviour	New alternative behaviour
Focus on self to assess social performance	Focus on others. Be really curious and interested about what others think and how they behave.
Try to control anxiety symptoms	Welcome anxiety. Give anxiety permission to stay
Avoid eye-contact with others	Increase eye contact with others.
Mentally rehearse what is being said before it is said.	Speak without thinking and assess what actually happens.
Try to control facial expressions by focussing on face.	Focus externally and give permission for your face to do whatever it chooses.
Focus on appearance	Focus on what you like about other people's appearance.

Table 14b. Potential behavioural experiments for social anxiety

Current behaviour	New alternative behaviour
Have a safe person with you when going to social situations.	Go to a social event alone.
Drink alcohol before going out to relax.	Go to social events in a state of sobriety.
Sit close to an exit so as to escape unnoticed.	Sit in a central area where you will have to move past people to leave the situation.
Hold onto or lean onto something supportive to hide shaking or trembling.	Allow hands to tremble. Allow others to see. Use external focus to assess what actually happens.
Use heavy makeup to avoid others noticing blushing or cover face with hair.	Use less make-up. Give permission for self to blush. Allow blushing experience to come and go. Use external focus to assess what actually happens.
Go to the toilet before going out (related to fear of using lavatories and others overhearing lavatory use.) Not being able to urinate at a urinal.	Use a lavatory in a public building. Use the lavatory while others are there. If male urinate in a urinal while other men are there. If unable to urinate wait for as long as is necessary.

Table 14c. Potential behavioural experiments for social anxiety

Current behaviour	New alternative behaviour
Carry a bottle of water (to help with a dry mouth).	Leave water at home. Let dry mouth be there.
Wear light clothing, fan self or stand near a window or a doorway to prevent over-heating. Alternatively wear more clothes to conceal sweating	Wear normal clothing and stand in a warmer part of the room. Use external focus to assess what actually happens.
Avoid conversations with people	Start a conversation with a new person. Introduce yourself to them, by telling them your name.
Have stories ready to put on an act of social competence and to have something interesting to say.	Go through a social event without telling stories or offering an acting performance. Practice active listening instead, using external focus.
Drink out a bottle rather than a glass to avoid others noticing shaking hands.	Drink out of a glass. If hands shake give permission for this to occur. Focus externally to assess what actually happens.
Stand in a corner to keep a low profile.	Stand in a more prominent position where you are likely to interact with more people.

Table 14d. Potential behavioural experiments for social anxiety

Current behaviour	New alternative behaviour
Keep conversations as short as possible to avoid revealing anything that could be self-incriminating	Offer up some information about yourself that you would not normally. Assess what others reactions are.
Have tissue ready to wipe hands to conceal sweaty hands.	Shake hands with somebody without wiping your hands first with tissues.
Have excuses about why you need to leave pre-planned and ready.	Go to events without any pre-planning.
Use diazepam or beta-blockers before social events e.g., business meetings.	Go to business meetings or social events without using medication.
Carry a supply of diazepam just in case.	Leave medication at home
Text instead of speaking to somebody in person	Speak to the person or telephone them rather than text

Table 15. Behavioural experiment sheet

Describe old behaviour or safety behaviour.

Monitor self for signs of anxiety

Describe new behaviour.

Drop monitoring.

How will you carry out new behaviour?

If I am aware that I am becoming anxious I will focus on accepting my anxiety and give it permission to be there.

Predictions about what will happen when you drop the safety behaviour. Write down as many scenarios as possible.

Probably nothing as they are my good friends and know me pretty well.
My anxiety may surprise me and I could look awkward and say something silly or embarrassing.

Carry out new behaviour and write down what actually happened here.

I became anxious at one point when there was a silence in the conversation. My stomach went over and I started to feel quite awkward. I focussed on allowing my anxiety to be there and my anxiety eased slightly. After a short while one of my friends started talking about another subject.

What did you learn from this process?
How likely are you to carry out this new behaviour again?

My anxiety passed very quickly and no one seemed concerned about it. Allowing anxiety to be there helps me feel slightly more relaxed.

Table 15. Behavioural experiment sheet

Describe old behaviour or safety behaviour.

Focus on myself to assess how I am coming across

Describe new behaviour.

Focus externally. I will place my attention as much as possible on my friends and the environment. I will look at my friends and listen to what they say.

How will you carry out new behaviour?

If I find myself going back to looking in at myself, I will immediately return to externally focusing once more.

Predictions about what will happen when you drop the safety behaviour. Write down as many scenarios as possible.

Looking at my friends will make them feel uncomfortable and my anxiety will increase.
I may feel less anxious as I will not be focussing on myself.
I had a memory from the past of someone saying "What are you staring at?" and this sticks in my mind.

Carry out new behaviour and write down what actually happened here.

I found that I felt much less anxious. At times I felt that I was going back into myself but pushed myself to focus externally.

What did you learn from this process?
How likely are you to carry out this new behaviour again?

It is much easier than I thought and I felt that I was much more associated in my body. I am going to keep using this going forwards.

Behavioural experiment sheet

Describe old behaviour or safety behaviour.

Describe new behaviour.

How will you carry out new behaviour?

Predictions about what will happen when you drop the safety behaviour. Write down as many scenarios as possible.

Carry out new behaviour and write down what actually happened here.

What did you learn from this process? How likely are you to carry out this new behaviour again?

Behavioural experiment sheet

Describe old behaviour or safety behaviour.

Describe new behaviour.

How will you carry out new behaviour?

Predictions about what will happen when you drop the safety behaviour. Write down as many scenarios as possible.

Carry out new behaviour and write down what actually happened here.

What did you learn from this process? **How likely are you to carry out this new behaviour again?**

Behavioural experiment sheet

Describe old behaviour or safety behaviour.

Describe new behaviour.

How will you carry out new behaviour?

Predictions about what will happen when you drop the safety behaviour. Write down as many scenarios as possible.

Carry out new behaviour and write down what actually happened here.

What did you learn from this process? **How likely are you to carry out this new behaviour again?**

Behavioural experiment sheet

Describe old behaviour or safety behaviour.

Describe new behaviour.

How will you carry out new behaviour?

Predictions about what will happen when you drop the safety behaviour. Write down as many scenarios as possible.

Carry out new behaviour and write down what actually happened here.

What did you learn from this process? How likely are you to carry out this new behaviour again?

Behavioural experiment sheet

Describe old behaviour or safety behaviour.

Describe new behaviour.

How will you carry out new behaviour?

Predictions about what will happen when you drop the safety behaviour. Write down as many scenarios as possible.

Carry out new behaviour and write down what actually happened here.

What did you learn from this process? How likely are you to carry out this new behaviour again?

Chapter summary

Behavioural experiments with social anxiety

- Behavioural experiments are very helpful for challenging safety behaviours that maintain symptoms of social anxiety.
- Completing a behavioural experiment involves you making a prediction about what you think is going to occur, doing it, and then finding out what actually happens.

22 An easy way to reprogram the subcortical mind

Summarising once more. For many individuals there is a distinct journey that their social anxiety has taken. In many cases – but not all - a painful childhood experience occurs, for example;

- Other children pointing out or noticing a physiological response such as blushing.
- A sports coach humiliating a child or making jokes about a child in front of his or her teammates.
- A child's mind going blank when asked a question by a teacher or getting an answer wrong in front of a teacher.
- Being laughed at or ridiculed by others.
- Being told off by authority figures in front of peers

Social anxiety may also be developed through a process of social learning, for example, as a result of being brought up by a socially anxious parent or by learning to fear social events through assimilation, e.g., watching parental figures become anxious before social events, see chapter 4.

Following initial traumatic experiences or early learning experiences the threat perception centre - while doing its job properly - looks out for environmental or social cues that may be connected to similar past traumatic situations. If a potential cue to a threat is noticed the threat perception centre immediately gives the all clear for production of an anxiety response. The individual recognises his or her physiological response (to anxiety) in a social situation, and intuitively attempts to conceal or control it. The individual monitors his or her anxiety levels and focuses on the self, in an attempt to reduce the threat exposed by the social interaction. While doing this many individuals begin to utilise safety behaviours such as trying to avoid eye contact, saying very little, etc. These behaviours become engrained and automatic over time through a process of negative reinforcement. As time progresses, this leads to a gradual erosion of confidence in social situations. Ultimately, the whole process can have a negative impact on friendships, intimate relationships, and in more extreme cases lead to individuals feeling lonely and emotionally isolated.

Starting to take charge of your life

Some or all of the above may be relevant to you in your situation, but the starting point of taking charge of your life will be to **desensitise** yourself to your own fear reactions.

Desensitising means approaching a problem gradually in order to teach the body how to become less affected by it. It is not unlike being inoculated against a disease. When you are inoculated small amounts of a virus or bacteria (generally inactive) will be injected into you or swallowed by you to teach your body how to cope with more serious strains of a virus or bacteria that you could be exposed to later on. Similarly, desensitisation could also be thought of as "behavioural inoculation." Dealing with very mild challenges initially, will help your mind and body cope with more serious challenges later on.

To complete desensitisation you will need to write down all of the situations that you have been avoiding. You will then need to grade each item on your list in terms of the level of anxiety you will experience when approaching the feared situation. Rate the most frightening item on your list as a ten and then compare each other situation to it giving each item on your list an anxiety score out of ten.

It is always best to start with approaching social situations, that produce the lowest anxiety levels, (an example list is shown on the next page). In each case it is very important that you accept your feelings while doing it (see processing emotions chapter). You will also need to be mindful that when completing items on your list that you do this without using any additional subtle safety behaviours, such as holding your breath, distracting yourself, etc.

Do not move onto higher anxiety evoking things on your list until your anxiety about completing things lower down on your list has reduced significantly or is easily tolerated.

I have placed a typical social avoidance list below.

Social avoidance list

1. Meet old friends for coffee (2)
2. Have lunch with fellow academics (4)
3. Agree to join a university committee (7)
4. Join a hockey club (7)
5. Attend a University social get together (8)
6. Present a lecture at another UK university (9)
7. Present a lecture at a conference abroad (10)
8. Go out on a date (10)

To assist yourself you could recognise that each social event that you have been avoiding can be broken down into much smaller units. If safety behaviours are difficult to drop these can also be approached using **systematic** desensitisation. Systematic basically means that you have a plan connected to it. I have placed a few examples of systematic desensitisation sheets on the next few pages. These will give you an idea of what I mean.

Using exposure sheets

Exposure is part of a process of desensitisation. When you use desensitisation you will need to stay in anxiety provoking situations until your anxiety is very easy to tolerate. To assist with your learning process you could assess your anxiety level before, during, and after the situation (see table 20). After you have completed exposure think to yourself about what you have learnt from your experience. This will further embed your experiential learning, (learning by experiencing).

NB: If you find that your anxiety does not reduce using desensitisation, don't persist with this approach. This might mean that you have unprocessed memories or traumatic experiences that need attention or working through. Unprocessed memories or traumas can often be a contributory factor to anticipatory anxiety in the present time mode. If this is the case, I recommend that that you don't try to work on these memories on your own. You will be better off working with a therapist.

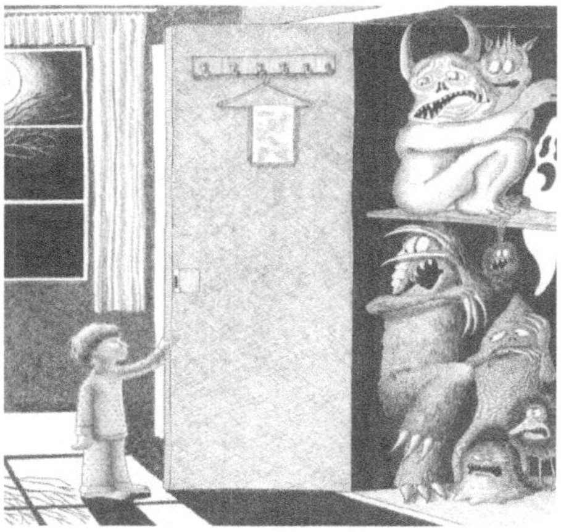

"You won't find out what actually happens unless you come out of the wardrobe!"

Table 16. Example of systematic desensitisation sheet

Overall target situation, object, or behaviour for desensitisation
Having lunch with fellow academics

Individual target area for desensitisation	Predicted distress level 0 to 10
Have lunch with a trusted fellow academic outside of the University campus, in order to discuss a research paper.	1
Use external focus with trusted colleague	2
Go to canteen when other staff members are there. Buy a drink and take it back to my office.	2
Buy a drink when other staff members are there and join staff members for 5 minutes.	2
Buy some food. Join fellow academics near the end of their lunch for five minutes.	3
Go down for lunch when other academics are there. Stay for twenty minutes.	3.5
Go to lunch part way through - Stay for thirty minutes	3.5
Go down for lunch with fellow academics. Stay until the end of lunch	4

Table 17. Example of systematic desensitisation sheet

Overall target situation, object, or behaviour for desensitisation

Offering up information about myself. Part of challenging my fear of vulnerability. Working towards being more open with colleagues.

Individual target area for desensitisation	Predicted distress level 0 to 10
Tell a trusted person something about myself that she does not know. Assess reaction.	2
Tell my line manager that I am working to try to reduce my social anxiety.	2.5
Tell one of my colleagues about a private 'safe' fear I have about offering lectures. Assess his reaction.	3
Have a chat with one of the administration staff and tell her what I am doing at the weekend.	3
Tell my most trusted colleague how I am feeling about something.	4
Tell a fellow academic one of my professional doubts about my research	5
Be open about a minor problem in front of two colleagues	6.5
Be open about a minor problem in front of a group of colleagues	7

Systematic desensitisation sheet

Overall target situation, object, or behaviour for desensitisation

Individual target area for desensitisation	**Predicted distress level 0 to 10**

Table 18. Exposure sheet

Time/date	**Situation**	**Anxiety before (0 - 10 where 10 is max)**	**Anxiety during (0 - 10 where 10 is max)**	**Anxiety after (0 - 10 where 10 is max)**	**What did I learn?**

Systematic desensitisation sheet

Overall target situation, object, or behaviour for desensitisation

Individual target area for desensitisation	**Predicted distress level 0 to 10**

Table 18. Exposure sheet

Time/date	Situation	Anxiety before (0 - 10 where 10 is max)	Anxiety during (0 - 10 where 10 is max)	Anxiety after (0 - 10 where 10 is max)	What did I learn?

Systematic desensitisation sheet

Overall target situation, object, or behaviour for desensitisation

Individual target area for desensitisation	**Predicted distress level 0 to 10**

Table 18. Exposure sheet

Time/date	Situation	Anxiety before (0 - 10 where 10 is max)	Anxiety during (0 - 10 where 10 is max)	Anxiety after (0 - 10 where 10 is max)	What did I learn?

Systematic desensitisation sheet

Overall target situation, object, or behaviour for desensitisation

Individual target area for desensitisation	**Predicted distress level 0 to 10**

Table 18. Exposure sheet

Time/date	Situation	Anxiety before (0 - 10 where 10 is max)	Anxiety during (0 - 10 where 10 is max)	Anxiety after (0 - 10 where 10 is max)	What did I learn?

Systematic desensitisation sheet

Overall target situation, object, or behaviour for desensitisation

Individual target area for desensitisation	**Predicted distress level 0 to 10**

Table 18. Exposure sheet

Time/date	Situation	Anxiety before (0 - 10 where 10 is max)	Anxiety during (0 - 10 where 10 is max)	Anxiety after (0 - 10 where 10 is max)	What did I learn?

Chapter summary

An easy way to reprogram the threat perception centre

- To desensitise yourself to your feelings of anxiety make a list of all of the things that you have been avoiding.

- Gradually work your way through the list approaching the item which evokes the least anxiety first making room for your feelings at all times.

23 What did you make of that?

A process that you can use as you reprogram the primitive part of your brain and to further embed the results of your new experiences is to ask yourself what you have learnt.

A reflective process brings more useful thoughts to the front of your mind and into conscious awareness. I will give an example from Melissa once more. Initially, when the model of approaching anxiety was covered with her, Melissa was slightly hesitant about applying it. Her prediction was that her anxiety would at best say the same or it would become more intense. After initially producing some anxiety artificially by engaging in worrying thoughts Melissa then began to practice making room for and accepting her feelings.

Melissa reported that her symptoms of anxiety were initially a 7 out of 10, (where 10 would be the most intense her anxiety could be). After one minute of focussing on her feelings and accepting them she found that her anxiety had reduced to a 5. After two minutes her anxiety had reduced to a 2. When the exercise was complete Melissa felt quite shocked at the results. She had never imagined that this type of approach would reduce her symptoms of anxiety.

A reflective process after completing this exercise helped Melissa bring new more accurate ideas to her awareness. Through reflection she recognised that;

- The counter-intuitive approach worked in her session at least.
- That what she thought would happen did not happen.
- That by trying something new she felt a sense of hope
- That it was highly likely that the same approach would work outside of sessions also.

It was important to help Melissa to reflect on this process as much as possible because the brain does not automatically review and revise. In fact, it seems that it can continue to repeat patterns of behaviour, even when behaviours are outdated or no longer work effectively.

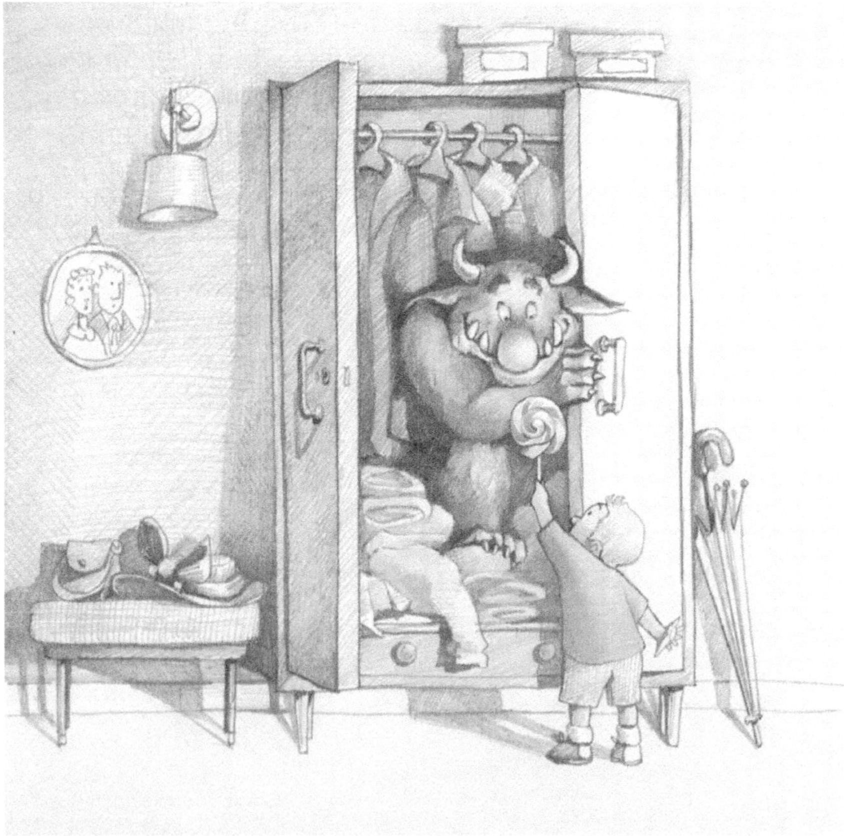

Chapter summary
What did you make of that?

- Asking reflective questions stimulates cognitive processes that can aid your learning experience.

- Bringing ideas into awareness such as what you thought might happen, what actually happened, and what you learnt will give you an opportunity to challenge thoughts that lie in the background of your mind creating a negative influence.

- Reflective processes encourage the brain to review and revise outdated, inefficient, and inaccurate thinking processes.

24 How to prevent relapse

To reduce relapse problems with our clients we began to use an idea that we referred to as the 'Law of Opposites' (Ridgeway & Manning, 2008). With this approach, at the end of treatment we would ask our clients to think about all the ideas that they might forget about or the behaviours that they could once again employ if they wanted to return to their original pre-therapy position. We encouraged our clients to make their list as exhaustive as possible.

Gregory's list is shown on the following page (see table 19). On reflection, the main thing Gregory noticed was that as he had become more open with trusted others, they too had become more open with him. He discovered that others he thought were ultra-confident experienced anxiety too. This knowledge affected him quite profoundly and led to Gregory feeling very differently about himself. Instead of viewing his anxiety as a threat he was now much more willing to recognise and appreciate that his body was creating a preparatory response for him. When he viewed his anxiety in this way it no longer felt as though anxiety was his enemy. When he approached situations such as chairing meetings he took his anxiety with him. Generally, he noticed that his anxiety only rose in the early stages of meetings, but as soon as he embraced it, it began to disappear.

Table 19. Law of opposites approach

Previous approach	New approach
Avoid difficult situations	Approach difficult situations
Put on a performance	Be myself. If I'm happy I'm happy, if I'm sad I'm sad.
Perceive anxiety symptoms as threatening. Try to escape from them	Perceive anxiety as part of the body that is trying to help me. Embrace symptoms.
Take medication before meetings	Do not use medication
Try to hide symptoms of anxiety	If I become anxious – Let the feelings be there. Anxiety is a healthy normal reaction
Disclose as little as possible about myself	Disclose information about myself to others who I trust. Disclose at the right time with the right people helps to break down barriers and can improve relationships.

A useful idea is to get your list out on a regular basis to assess if there is any slippage back to your previous way of approaching your symptoms. Keeping a log that documents your journey with social anxiety may also prove useful. You will then be able to look back over this log at a future point in time if you need to quickly revise or recap on approaches that worked for you.

Chapter summary

How to prevent relapse

- If you discontinue using the techniques learnt in this book there is an increased likelihood of relapse.
- Become aware of the risk factors involved in relapse by using the "Law of Opposites" exercise.
- Regularly look at your risk factors and if you notice any slippage back to your old positon then put your counter-intuitive strategies in place.
- Keep a log of your experiences. Reflect on the result of positive changes.

28

Conclusion

You have now come to the end of this CBT book for social anxiety. In this book we have covered some of the main areas that are covered in CBT sessions for social anxiety. If you decide to attend CBT sessions at some point, hopefully you will have some idea of the types of things that will be discussed.

If you decide to see a CBT therapist your therapist will ask you about what problems in particular you would like to work on. Picking a particular problem and writing down your thoughts and feelings about this problem will be very helpful, as you and your therapist will then be able to discuss it. You may also note down situations that lead to you feeling distressed, and how you think, feel, and behave in these situations.

You may also need to be aware before you start your CBT that it will involve you changing a) the way that you think, b) how you relate to your feelings and c) how you behave. Changing the way that you think, feel and behave can be very difficult, due to habitual behaviour.

Much of the time we can find ourselves falling into repetitive loops when we become highly emotional. Many of us use the same habitual behaviours over and over again to deal with our emotions in certain situations, even when we know that our strategies don't work. As I mentioned earlier traditional neuroscience suggests that the seat of habit formation can be found in the basal ganglia, a sub-cortical region of the brain. When we become distressed, states of high emotional arousal lead to primitive brain areas located in the sub-cortical area taking a central role. These primitive brain areas are governed by habitual behaviour, which tends to be automatic, inflexible, and rule-based.

Habitual behaviour is generally thought to operate outside of conscious awareness and we revert to this quite strongly when under stress.

CBT can bring your habitual behaviour to your awareness so that you can choose to do things differently. Breaking habitual cycles is not very easy because they are neurologically wired in. However, with repetition, your new positive habits can be stored in your basal ganglia alongside your old habits.

...Very best of luck with your therapy...

Advice for loved ones

If you live with someone with social anxiety you will be aware that this can cause difficulties in several areas, but especially within family life or within relationships. Your loved one may want to avoid many different types of social situations which can lead to reduced opportunities for you or other family members to socialise as you might ideally like. What to you may feel like an exciting social opportunity is likely to feel like daunting experiences for your loved one with social anxiety.

At times there may be upcoming social situations that your loved one has to attend for one reason or another. When this occurs you may recognise increased tension in the household preceding these events. Ideally, you will have read this book and understand the distress that your loved one experiences is not about his or her relationship with you. Individuals with social anxiety have a heightened fear of being judged. As such, they are likely to experience distress preceding social events (through worry), during social events (through self-monitoring), and after social events (through a process of rumination). When you think about the level of suffering that your loved one is likely to experience it makes perfect sense that your loved one will want to avoid these types of events. Avoidance is not an ideal solution, however. As you may already realise that if your loved one does manage to avoid social situations then he or she is also more likely to suffer from low self-esteem, loneliness, reduced confidence, and possibly low mood. In this respect, your loved feels pain regardless of what he or she does.

With the above in mind, it will be important to encourage your loved one to utilise the strategies contained in this book. Practicing strategies with you will help you to help your loved one to drop safety behaviours and form a different relationship with feelings. It is important to recognise that although your loved one may be socially anxious, it will be more beneficial for you not to become complicit in your loved ones avoidance strategies, and thus is very important that you continue with your own social life accordingly. Carrying on with your own social life will make it more difficult for your loved one to stay within his or her trapped position.

Luckily, there are many things that you can do to help your loved one when they are feeling distressed about upcoming social events. One of the most effective strategies is systematic desensitisation. People with social anxiety prefer to spend time with people who they know, and who they perceive are accepting. Gradually, introducing new people one or two at a time is likely to be the most effective approach in this respect. Encouraging your loved one to talk with you about the strategies that they have read about in this book and what he or she is going to do differently can offer a useful outlet for your loved one to learn.

If your loved one is anxious before a social event it will generally be a good idea to drop all rationalising and reassurance preceding the event. Individuals in a state of anxiety rarely hear or process rational information. Instead it will be far more effective to encourage your loved one to attend social events while validating his or her feelings. Let your loved one know that they are feeling anxious, that there are good reasons for this anxiety, and that you are fully accepting of his or her anxiety. For example, "I know that this is a very difficult situation for you, and that you feel uncomfortable about this. It's not easy and I know that you would rather not go." Speaking in this way does not give permission for your loved one to avoid a social situation, but it does acknowledge how difficult it is for your loved one. A general rule of thumb is that gentle encouragement is the best approach for somebody that is feeling anxious, rather than frustration, shouting, or showing anger.

Appendix

Regulatory organisations in the UK

British Association of Cognitive and Behavioural Psychotherapists
Imperial House
Hornby Street
Bury
Lancashire
BL9 5BN
Tel: 0161 705 4304 Fax: 0161 705 4306
Email: babcp@babcp.com

British Association for Counselling & Psychotherapy
BACP House
15 St John's Business Park
Lutterworth
LE17 4HB
Tel 01455 883300

British Psychological Society
St Andrews House
48 Princess Road East
Leicester
LE1 7DR
United Kingdom
Tel: +44 (0)116 254 9568
Fax: +44 (0)116 227 1314
Email: **enquiries@bps.org.uk**

Health & Care Professional Council
Park House
184 Kennington Park Road,
London
SE11 4BU,
0300 500 6184

References and additional reading

Arnsten, A, Raskind, M. Taylor, F, & Connor, D. *Neurobiology of Stress (*2015). The effects of stress exposure on prefrontal cortex: Translating basic research into successful treatments for post-traumatic stress disorder, pages 89–99

Bandura, A., (1977). *Social Learning Theory*. Prentice-Hall.

Beck, J. (2011) *Cognitive Behavior Therapy: Second Edition – Basics and Beyond.* The Guildford Press.

Butler, G., (2009). *Overcoming Social Anxiety & Shyness.* Robinson

Cabral, R & Nardi E . *(2012).* Anxiety and inhibition of panic attacks within translational and prospective research contexts. *Trends in Psychiatry*

Clark, D.M., (1986) A cognitive approach to panic: *Behaviour Research and Therapy*, 24: 461-470

Clark, D.M., & Wells, A (1995). A cognitive model of social phobia. In *Social Phobia – Diagnosis, Assessment, and Treatment* (eds R. G. Heimberg, M. R. Liebowitz, D. Hope, et al), pp. 69–93. New York: Guilford.

Debiec J., & Sullivan, R. (2014). Intergenerational transmission of emotional trauma through amygdala-dependent mother-to-infant transfer of specific fear. *PNAS*, DOI: 10.1073/pnas.1316740111

Golman, D., (1996) .Emotional intelligence: Why it can matter more than IQ. Bloomsbury

Guzmán, Y., Tronson, N., Jovasevic, K., Sato, K., Guedea, A., Mizukami, H., Nishimori, K., & Radulovic. J. (2013) Fear-enhancing effects of septal oxytocin receptors. *Nature Neuroscience*, 2013; DOI: 10.1038/nn.3465

Greenberger, D., & Padesky, C. (1995). *Mind Over Mood: Change How You Feel by Changing the Way That You Think.* Guildford Press Kennerley, H., (2009).

Kennerley, H., (2009). *Overcoming anxiety: A self-help guide using cognitive behavioural techniques*. Robinson
Kinman, G & Grant, L. (2010). Exploring Stress Resilience in Trainee Social Workers: The Role of Emotional and Social Competencies. *British Journal of Social Work*. 10.1093/bjsw/bcq088

Krusemark, E & Li. W., (2012). Enhanced Olfactory Sensory Perception of Threat in Anxiety: An Event-Related fMRI Study (2012). *Chemosensory Perception*, 5 (1): 37 DOI: 10.1007/s12078-011-9111-7

LeDoux JE[1], Iwata J, Cicchetti P, Reis DJ. Different projections of the central amygdaloid nucleus mediate autonomic and behavioral correlates of conditioned fear (1988). *J Neurosci.* Jul;8(7):2517-29.

Logue, M.W., Bauver, S.R., Kremen, W.S., Franz, C.E., Eisen, S.A., Tsuang, M.T., Grant, MD., & Lyons, M.J., (2011). Evidence of Overlapping Genetic Diathesis of Panic Attacks and Gastrointestinal Disorders in a Sample of Male Twin (2011).*Twin Res Hum Gene*t. Feb; 14(1): 16–24. doi: 10.1375/twin.14.1.16

McIlrath, D & Huitt, W. The teaching-learning process: A discussion of models. *Educational Psychology Interactive*. Valdosta, GA: Valdosta State University. Retrieved 2016 from http://www.edpsycinteractive.org/papers/modeltch.html

Moorey S[1] (2010). The six cycles maintenance model: Growing a "vicious flower" for depression. Behaviour and Cognitive Psychotherapy. Mar;38(2):173-84.

Moulding, Richard, Coles, Meredith E., Abramowitz, Jonathan S., Alcolado,Gillian M., Alonso, Pino, Belloch, Amparo, Bouvard, Martine, Clark, David A., Doron, Guy, Fernández-Álvarez, Hector, García-Soriano, Gemma, Ghisi, Marta, Gómez, Beatriz, Inozu, Mujgan, Radomsky, Adam S., Shams, Giti, Sica, Claudio, Simos, Gregoris & Wong, Wing (2014). Part 2. They scare because we care: the relationship between obsessive intrusive thoughts and appraisals and control strategies across 15 cities., *Journal of obsessive-compulsive and related disorders*, vol. 3, no. 3, pp. 280-291.

Rachman, S., Coughtrey, Shafran, R & Radomsky, A., (2015). *The Oxford Guide to the Treatment of Mental Contamination.* The Oxford University Press.

Seger, C.A., (2011). A critical review of habit learning and the Basal ganglia. *Front Syst Neuroscience*, Aug 30;5:66.

Teachman, B., Marker, C & Clerkin, E. (2010). Catastrophic misinterpretations as a predictor of symptom change during treatment for panic disorder (2010). *Consult Clin Psycho*l. 78(6): 964–973.

Veale, D., & Wilson, R., (2005). *Overcoming Obsessive Compulsive Disorder: A self-help guide using Cognitive Behavioral Techniques.*. Constable & Robinson Ltd

Wells, A. (1997) Cognitive Therapy of Anxiety Disorders: A Practice Manual and Conceptual Guide. Wiley.

Wilson, R., & Veale, D. (2009). *Overcoming Health Anxiety.* Robinson

Glossary

Academics - Academics spend a lot of time studying or researching specialist subjects at institutions like universities.

Abdominal breathing – Processing of breathing which involves relaxing the abdomen and taking in air to the bottom of the lungs.

Amygdala – Small area of brain tissue within the limbic system, responsible for activating the body's fight-flight-or-freeze response.

Anxiety – An emotion which is experienced when the body is moving into a prepared state to deal with a potential threat.

Automatic responses – Responses which occur automatically/outside of conscious awareness.

Behavioural strategies – Making an adjustment to your behaviour and monitoring the impact of resulting changes.

Catastrophic misinterpretation – A frightening and exaggerated thought connected to magnification of perceived stimuli.

Catecholamines – Chemical messengers used by cells to communicate with one and other.

Cognitive distortions – Thinking patterns that distort perception of reality.

Cognitive models – Ways of explaining how psychological distress is maintained.

Cognitive interventions – Strategies based on changing mental reactions.

Conditioned response – A response that occurs automatically as a result of repeated actions towards particular stimuli.

Coping strategies – Strategies that have been of some assistance in reducing distress.

Core beliefs – Strongly held beliefs about the self.

Counter-intuitive – Ideas which we would not naturally gravitate towards.

Default response – An automatic response based on previous experiences and past conditioning.

Desensitising - Gradually being able to tolerate a feeling by staying in a situation until the feeling feels more bearable.

Diazepam – A medication often prescribed as a muscle relaxant.

Dissociation – A mental and physical state where an individual feels a loss of connection with his or her body.

Distraction – A process that individuals use to avoid experiencing painful emotions.

Emotional reference point – A mechanism used by babies who look towards caregivers to determine how they might react at an emotional level.

Experiential – A process of experiencing through the senses.

External focus – Placing one's attention onto one's external environment.

Habitual behaviours – Behaviours that we are inclined to do because we have do because we have done them so many times before.

Holistic – Multiple process connected together working in parallel.

Hyperventilation – A process of rapid shallow breathing where an individual breathes out too much carbon dioxide.

Hypothesis – An idea based on scientific theory.

Intrusive thoughts – Thoughts that enter awareness uninvited. These thought are usually accompanied by heightened emotion.

Intrusive thoughts – Thoughts that enter awareness uninvited. These thought are usually accompanied by heightened emotion.

Mindfulness – A process of staying in the present moment, bringing conscious awareness back to the present, and deliberately moving away from thoughts about the past or the future.

Mood regulation – An ability to have some management of one's feelings.

Negative automatic thoughts - Thoughts in the background of the mind that have the potential to keep individuals emotionally distressed.

Negative reinforcement – A process of repeated behaviour in which negative emotion is reduced leading to greater likelihood of the same future behaviour.

Neocortex – Highly developed area of the mind responsible for logical, rational and analytical thinking.

Phobic response – An automatic response associated with heightened anxiety, connected to a specific trigger or cue.

Plasticity – The brains ability to repair itself and grow the more that it is used.

Prefrontal cortex – An area of the brain that acts as a relay between the subcortical regions of the brain and the neo-cortex. It is also responsible for dampening emotional reactions and quietening the mind.

Registered therapists – Registered therapists are members of professional bodies. Professional bodies are organisations that check out their therapists to make sure that they have the required training to do their jobs properly.

Rumination – A cognitive process which involves churning of thoughts connected to the self in the past over and over in the mind.

Safety behaviours - Behaviours utilised to reduce emotional distress in the short-term.

Self-fulfilling prophesy – When something occurs despite your very best attempts to prevent that particular thing occurring.

Self-perpetuating – A situation that is kept in place through its own actions.

Serotonin - A chemical messenger serotine plays a huge part in the body's overall physical and mental Functioning.

Subcortical regions – Brain areas located in the lower half of the brain.

Supressing emotions – An act of pushing down painful or upsetting feelings.

Threat Perception Centre – An area within the brain responsible to noticing stimuli associated with past fear or trauma.

Supressing emotions – An act of pushing down painful or upsetting feelings.

Threat Perception Centre – An area within the brain responsible to noticing stimuli associated with past fear or trauma.

Traumatic incidents – Events that have occurred in the past connected to highly distressing emotions.

Unprocessed memory - An experience that the mind has not fully dealt with.

Vicarious trauma - When people develop trauma responses as a result of observing other people's intense emotional reactions.

Common medications

Alprazolam – A benzodiazepine prescribed for panic, generalised anxiety, phobias, social anxiety, OCD

Amitriptyline – A tricyclic antidepressant

Atenolol – A beta-blocker prescribed for anxiety

Buspirone – A mild tranquiliser prescribed for generalised anxiety, OCD and panic

Chlordiazepoxide – A benzodiazepine prescribed for generalised anxiety, phobias

Citalopram – A selective serotonin reuptake inhibitor commonly prescribed for mixed anxiety and depression

Clomipramine – A tricyclic antidepressant

Clonazepam – A benzodiazepine prescribed for panic, generalised anxiety, phobias, social anxiety

Desipramine – A tricyclic anti-depressant

Diazepam – A benzodiazepine prescribed for generalised anxiety, panic, phobias

Doxepin – A tricyclic antidepressant

Duloxetine – A serotonin-norepinephrine reuptake inhibitor

Escitalopram Oxalate – A selective serotonin reuptake inhibitor

Fluoxetine - A selective serotonin reuptake inhibitor

Fluvoxamine – A selective serotonin reuptake inhibitor

Gabapentin – An anticonvulsant prescribed for generalised anxiety and social anxiety

Imipramine – A tri-cyclic antidepressant

Lorazepam – A benzodiazepine prescribed for generalised anxiety, panic, phobias

Nortriptyline – A tricyclic antidepressant

Oxazepam – A benzodiazepine prescribed for generalised anxiety, phobias

Paroxetine – A selective serotonin reuptake inhibitor

Phenelzine – A monoamine oxidase inhibitor

Pregabalin – An anticonvulsant prescribed for generalised anxiety disorder

Propanalol – A beta blocker prescribed for anxiety

Sertraline - A selective serotonin reuptake inhibitor

Tranylcypromine – A monoamine oxidase inhibitor

Valproate – An anti-convulsant prescribed for panic

Venlafaxine – A serotonin-norepinephrine reuptake inhibitor

Made in United States
Cleveland, OH
05 November 2026

47664325R00103